LES
MORE LIFE

Is Weight Loss Surgery Right For You?

Top 2 1 Questions You Need to Ask!

LESS WEIGHT MORE LIFE

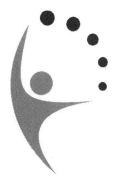

Is Weight Loss Surgery Right For You?

Top 2 I Questions You Need to Ask!

Thomas W. Clark, MS, MD, FACS

Board Certified Bariatric Surgeon and Bariatrician

Center for Weight Loss Success, PC

LESS WEIGHT MORE LIFE

Is Weight Loss Surgery
Right For You?

Top 21 Questions
You Need to Ask!

© 2012 Thomas W. Clark, MS, MD, FACS

Published by Adriel Publishing

Edited by Karol H. Clark, MSN, RN

FIRST EDITION

Printed in the U.S.A.

Cover design by Liz Lawless

ISBN-13: 978-1-939998-00-2

www.cfwls.com

Dedication

To anyone who wants to lose a considerable amount of weight and is considering making a healthy change in their life through one of the most effective tools available – weight loss surgery. It is an amazing journey and I dedicate this book to you as you make this very important and life changing decision. May this book help answer your questions as you determine what weight loss path is right for you. You deserve long term success, happiness, health and a life that fulfills your dreams.

I also dedicate this book to the thousands of amazing motivated people who have chosen me as their weight loss surgeon – I am honored. You and your long term success gives true meaning to what I do every day.

Life is what we do minute to minute and day to day...be sure to enjoy the journey along the way...

Dr. Thomas W. Clark

Disclaimer

Some of the information in this book is anecdotal opinions from the author after practicing extensively and exclusively in the field of bariatric surgery (performing nearly 4,000 primary weight loss surgery procedures) and bariatric medicine. Unless otherwise stated, statements are based upon his extensive clinical experience (and common sense) over the past 20 years specializing in bariatric surgery and bariatric medicine. The opinions of clients are theirs and were freely given.

Table of Contents

A Note from the Author

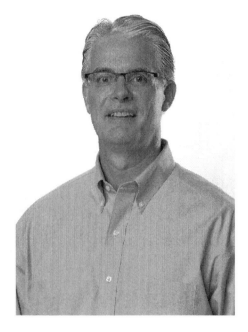

Thomas W. Clark, MS, MD, FACS

I am a board certified weight loss surgeon and bariatrician. I specialize in helping people who struggle with their weight. I not only help them lose it but keep it off for good. This significantly improves their health. I have been doing this successfully for nearly two decades. Helping people lose weight and understand how to keep it off is my mission in life. This gives meaning to what I do every day. It's amazing to see the transformation. I not only give people a new surgical "tool" to lose weight and improve their health quickly, but I provide them with a comprehensive step-by-step program so they not only lose weight but change their underlying habits. This ensures they enjoy their success *for life!*

I grew up on a farm outside of Buffalo, NY. I am used to hard work. I used what little money I had to put myself through school. I worked to make ends meet along with many student loans. When I finished college, I was like many people – I wasn't sure exactly what I wanted to do. I thought about medical school but knew that if I pursued that career, it would be an intense lifetime commitment and I wasn't sure I was ready. I loved working with my hands so I began working as a cabinet maker. After a couple of years, I decided to take the exam for medical school and did great. My medical school interviews went well and I began my pursuit of becoming a surgeon at Wake Forest University in NC. It's hard to believe now, but I completed my surgical residency nearly 20 years ago. During that time, I was trained to perform weight loss surgery. However, after residency, I thought I would focus on general surgery and never perform bariatric surgery again.

Once I began my surgical career in Virginia, I found a real need in the community and a desire within myself to help overweight individuals who were struggling with their health and unable to fully enjoy their lives. I began performing weight loss surgery and something amazing happened. I found a group of the most grateful individuals and families I had ever come in contact with.

In the 1990's, I decided to do something unheard of at the time – I chose to specialize exclusively in bariatric surgery. Over time, I found some of these grateful people began to regain their weight. They were frustrated and so was I. I realized that they regained their weight because the tool almost worked "too well". You see weight loss is inevitable after weight loss surgery (particularly during the first year) but if you don't understand how to use your new tool most effectively and change your underlying habits, you are potentially set up for long-term failure.

This began my quest to have the most comprehensive quality weight loss surgery program available *anywhere*. Over the past twenty years, I have been able to do just that. I have performed nearly 4,000 weight loss procedures, become board certified in bariatric medicine as well and developed a curriculum called *Weight Management University*™ and *Weight Management University for Weight Loss Surgery*™. The curriculum helps to ensure long term weight loss success for anyone who wants to lose 5 pounds or hundreds of pounds.

These programs work so well that I want to share them with surgeons, physicians, hospitals and patients everywhere. Now

I give clients not only a tool to lose weight through surgery, but teach them how to keep it off so they can get their life back and enjoy the things others sometimes take for granted. This has led me on a wonderful and fulfilling journey.

If you struggle with your weight, I welcome you to enhance your life journey by being the healthiest you can be. It starts with research into what's best for you. I hope this book proves to be your guide to not only answer the questions you have but also additional questions you should consider. This is a journey well worth taking and leads you to a fuller and healthier life, free of the disease called morbid obesity.

To receive Dr. Clark's free special report for successful weight loss, visit www.cfwls.com. You can also follow him on:

Twitter at www.twitter.com/docweightloss

Facebook at www.facebook.com/weightlossdrclark,

YouTube at www.youtube.com/docweightloss

And newly released in 2012, see Dr. Clark on his online weight loss TV station at www.DocWeightLoss.TV.

Foreword

A STORY WORTH READING

BY RHONDA HOFFMAN

The first on camera interview I did for surgical weight loss patients was 6 months after my surgery with Dr. Clark. I was still shy while sitting in front of a camera, (still feeling like the old image of myself, but not looking like that old image). The most vivid moment of that interview was when I was asked how I felt about the results of the surgery. I responded by honestly saying "I don't have my old life back, I have a better life." True at that time, but now that I am three years out from my surgery, I have to amend by saying "I have a fantastic life!" In fact, the most loving and brilliant action I ever took for myself in my life was having weight loss surgery at the age of 48.

My life now is nothing like I thought it was doomed too be at an early age. I vividly remember parents and family saying to me things like "You're a big boned girl", "It's in your genes" and "Not everyone can be thin."

I heard this for years from my family – all very large people. I thought it to be true and believed there was no way to change it. I was athletic in high school, to the point of all state honors for softball. I started at age 8 playing softball, (they always put the fat kid at catcher), the position stuck. I was the best "thick catcher in Iowa in 1980."

*A few years later, I watched as my mother died a slow painful death with type II diabetes. Then my father as well. For years, he fought congestive heart failure with type II diabetes. In 2009, I was home attending my father's funeral. I looked around the room at my remaining relatives – all where huge. My uncle was in a wheelchair with no left leg (a result of diabetes). My aunt was also in a wheelchair. She was obese and unable to walk. My brother was standing next to me, only one year older, and pushing 350 pounds and I was a size 20 myself, all dressed in black. At that very moment I thought, "**I need to save my life!** Just because I'm related to these people doesn't mean I need to be like them. **I'm taking control of my life now!**"*

I called my primary care physician to make an appointment even before I returned home from Iowa, I needed help. I could not fix it myself with my unsuccessful history of yo-yo weight loss attempts. After all, she had told me recently I was pre-diabetic myself. We discussed my failed weight loss attempts and I told her I wanted to try weight loss surgery. She was very positive and offered a list of doctors in the area. I had thought of weight loss surgery in the past, but it seemed to be a secret people rarely shared with others. I only knew one woman who'd had the surgery 10 years prior; a friend gave me her number to talk to her. I would have never guessed she previously weighed 318 pounds. She was a size 8, very attractive.

I got my list of Doc's and started making calls. I am very keen to reception, and I was on high alert to see how I was treated as a potential customer and patient. I chose Dr. Clark's practice. The decision was made. I had found my Doctor and the village of support I would call on throughout my "rebirth" at his all-encompassing facility. Now I had a strong foundation of knowledgeable, helpful staff and tools, to be successful in permanent weight loss for the rest of my life.

Although my insurance did not cover weight loss surgery, I knew this was what I had to do. I knew Dr. Clark was the surgeon I needed and his comprehensive program was the right thing for me. As they say, the rest is history.

In addition to getting healthy not to be understated, it's a fantastic feeling to feel good every day; I have discovered other *benefits along the way. I have had many more professional op-portunities arise, my social calendar is full of activities I never thought I would be able to do (I use to wish I could bike ride a 100 miles, in a day, now I can do it! No more wishing, I can do anything I want to do now and that's a fact.)*

I'm healthy and I even gained financially. I have saved a lot of money on medications, and doctors for all my related aliments due to obesity. I eat healthy and spend less. It's the best money I ever spent; I've gotten it back tenfold in living. The cost was long forgotten, because I have gained it back in so many other ways it would take a book to explain. Don't make any more excuses, take control of your life, and your body will respond beyond your wildest dreams.

Thanks for reading my story. I want people to know they too can have a fantastic life!

Rhonda

Rhonda Before Surgery

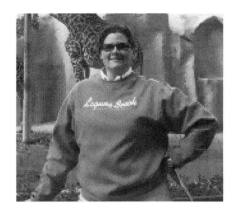

After

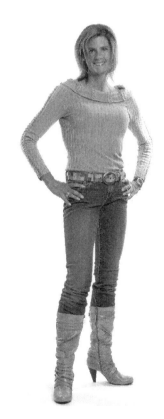

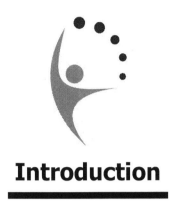

Introduction

Many common medical problems are directly associated with weight. Diabetes, high blood pressure, sleep apnea, high cholesterol, back and joint pain are just a few of them. These, and many others worsen as weight goes up. Almost all of them will improve (and many go away) as weight comes down.

Weight loss surgery is a personal decision that no one can (or should) make for you. It is your decision and yours alone. Weight loss surgery is a great option for massive weight loss, especially if you are motivated and understand that it is a tool to help you lose weight. However, you must learn how to use your new tool to lose weight for optimal long lasting results. If you do this, you are in for an amazing and rewarding journey.

Your decision to read this book indicates that you are motivated and want to make the best decision possible for your life and your health. Congratulations! In fact, the most successful people who undergo weight loss surgery are those that research what is available and ask the questions you are about to read about. If you are someone who views weight loss surgery as the "easy way out", "last resort" or "quick fix" you will definitely want to read further so you can understand that there is so much more to it than that. If you desire additional information, you can visit www.MyWeightLossSurgerySuccess.com for free videos that coincide with these chapters.

"The latest study based on a nationally representative sample of U.S. adults estimates that about 112,000 deaths are associated with obesity each year in the United States."[1] This is primarily due to the co-morbid conditions associated with obesity. In fact, according to a team of scientists supported in part by the National Institute on Aging (NIA), a component of the National Institutes of Health (NIH) of the Department of Health and Human Services, obesity threatens to lower the life expectancy for the average American by as much as 5 years.[2]

So what's five more years of life worth to you? It's a powerful question about a depressing reality in the United States and one that cannot be ignored.

While these statistics are devastating, there is hope. Aside from the "gimmick" weight loss programs and products that are pushed at you from every creative marketing angle, there are valuable programs that focus on all aspects of weight loss (nutrition, fitness and behavioral change) and that is what will give you long term results. In fact, if you are considering weight loss surgery, you must still make sure your surgical program includes these three facets so you not only lose the weight, but understand how to keep it off for life.

In this book, you will find a number of questions that are frequently asked. However, this book takes it one step further and investigates the questions you may not even know you need to ask. And that can be even more important when considering life changing opportunities. So, let's get started.

CHAPTER 1

What Are the Best Weight Loss Surgery Options Available Today?

Weight loss surgery has certainly evolved...thank goodness! Don't get me wrong, it is not without any risk but the procedures available today are much safer and more effective than procedures of the past.

This overview includes the three primary surgical procedures performed within the United States as of the publication of this book along with the advantages, risks and typical results and outcomes for each. These three procedures are the Sleeve Gastrectomy (also referred to as the Gastric Sleeve), the Laparoscopic Adjustable Gastric Banding (also referred to as LapBand® or Realize Band®) and the Laparoscopic Gastric Bypass.

Sleeve Gastrectomy:

The Sleeve Gastrectomy is a newer laparoscopic weight loss surgical procedure in which a small "sleeve-shaped" stomach is created. Approximately 75% of the "stretchy" portion of the stomach is removed. This also removes the portion of the stomach that makes the hormone ghrelin. Ghrelin is a hormone which makes you feel hungry. The remaining "sleeve" of the stomach is about the size and shape of a medium banana. Because anatomy remains normal, this procedure can be considered for people with less weight to lose (50-60 lbs. overweight).

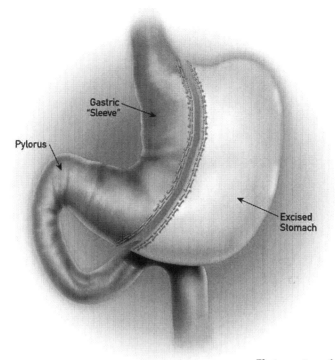

Photo courtesy of
Ethicon Endo-Surgery Inc.

Advantages:

- The portion of the stomach that produces ghrelin (a hormone that stimulates hunger) is removed.

- The stomach is reduced in volume, but otherwise tends to function normally.

- **No** "Dumping Syndrome" since the pylorus is preserved.

- **No** intestine is bypassed so there is little chance of nutritional deficiencies.

- **No** implanted device that requires adjusting.

- Procedure is performed laparoscopically most of the time.

- Often an outpatient procedure.

This procedure tends to work due to two major reasons:

1. You have a much smaller stomach and will feel full with eating only a small amount.

2. There is a decrease in the hormone ghrelin so that hunger is much easier to control.

The sleeve gastrectomy was originally developed as the 1st stage of a 2 stage procedure (patients would undergo a conversion of the sleeve gastrectomy to a bypass procedure). However, it was found to work so well on its own that most patients did not need (or want) to go through with the next stage.

This surgery cannot be reversed (i.e. once that part of the stomach is gone…it is gone).

Risks:

Obesity, age, and other diseases increase your risks from any surgery. Below are identified risks related to surgery and the sleeve gastrectomy procedure based upon national averages:

- Risk of death is 1:500-1,000

- Leaks (1-2%)

- Infection (2%)

- Blood Clot/Pulmonary Embolus (1%)

- Nausea/vomiting

- Peptic ulcer disease

- Formation of gallstones due to rapid weight loss

- Stricture (1%)

Some of these problems may require further surgical intervention.

Typical Results and Outcomes:

Weight loss outcomes are tracked closely at the Center for Weight Loss Success. We are proud that outcomes here generally out-perform national averages. The average best weight loss for this procedure is 65-70% of a client's excess body weight (i.e. if someone is 100 lbs. over their ideal body weight, average weight loss outcomes would be 65-70 lbs.).

A weight loss of only about 40% of excess body weight will often show significant improvement in many other medical problems:

- Many Type 2 diabetics will get off of their medications

- Hypertensive clients will have improvement or resolution of their hypertension

- Sleep apnea almost always improves

- Cholesterol improvement in most clients

- Arthritic symptoms improve

Laparoscopic Adjustable Gastric Banding (LapBand® or Realize Band®):

The FDA approved adjustable gastric banding surgery in June, 2001. However, it was developed in the 1980's and has been used in Europe since 1993. In terms of surgical procedures for weight loss, this is the least invasive procedure.

Laparoscopic adjustable gastric banding involves applying a band around the upper part of the stomach. As a result, this creates a small gastric pouch at the top of the stomach, with a small opening to the rest of the stomach. The band is made of an inflatable silastic ring that controls the flow of food from the small pouch to the rest of your digestive system. With this surgery, there is no cutting or stapling required for dividing the stomach.

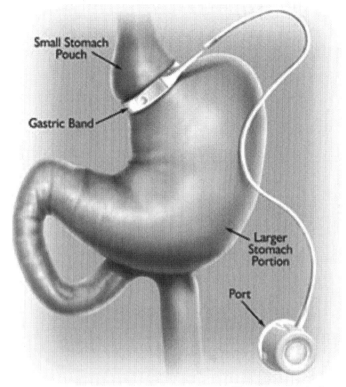

Small Stomach Pouch

Gastric Band

Larger Stomach Portion

Port

Photo courtesy of Allergan

In addition to the band, a small port is connected by tubing to the inflatable ring around the stomach.

The port is secured just beneath the skin where fluid can be injected or withdrawn to inflate or deflate (adjust) the band. This results in increasing or decreasing the size of the opening between the upper small gastric pouch and the lower portion of the stomach. The need for an adjustment is determined by the surgeon based upon weight loss and symptoms related to eating.

Like any tool, it can be used correctly or incorrectly. Used incorrectly (such as drinking high calorie liquids) you will have relatively poor weight loss or even weight gain. It is still diet, exercise, and behavior change which produce weight loss. **Thus, following your surgeon's recommendations is crucial to your overall success.**

Advantages:

- Risk of death is approximately 1:1000

- There is no division or re-routing of intestinal tract

- Minimal risk of malnutrition

- The procedure is considered reversible since the Band can be removed with minimally invasive technique if needed

The band is adjustable:

- Often performed under fluoroscopic guidance

- May require 4-6 adjustments during the first year (or more)

- Adjustments need to be checked yearly – **forever**

The band is effective with the following considerations:

- Weight loss success is directly related to:
  o close clinical follow-up
  o appropriate adjustments
  o exercise
  o diet and behavior modification

The potential **disadvantages** of laparoscopic adjustable gastric banding are as follows:

- Weight loss is typically slower when compared to other weight loss surgeries

- Adjustments are required throughout your lifetime

- Problems can develop secondary to the mechanical device

Risks:

Obesity, age, and other diseases increase your risks from any surgery. Below are identified risks related to surgery and the laparoscopic adjustable gastric banding procedure based upon national averages.

- Risk of death is 1:1000

9

- Infection (<1%)

- Blood Clot/Pulmonary Embolus (1%)

- Gastric pouch dilation potentially requiring further surgery (5%)

- Band slippage or migration often requiring further surgery (5%)

- Band erosion requiring further surgery for band removal (1%)

- Access port problem or tubing leak requiring further surgery

- Nausea/vomiting

- Peptic ulcer disease

- Formation of gallstones due to rapid weight loss

Some of these problems may require further surgical intervention.

Typical Results and Outcomes:

Following are expected results and outcomes based upon national averages:

- Average weight loss is 45-50% of excess body weight, but with aggressive diet and exercise changes you can lose almost all of your excess weight.

- A weight loss of only about 40% of excess body weight will often show significant improvement in many other medical problems:

  ○ Many of Type 2 diabetics will get off of medications

  ○ Hypertensive clients will have improvement or resolution of their hypertension

  ○ Sleep apnea almost always improves

  ○ Cholesterol improvement in most clients

  ○ Arthritic symptoms improve

Laparoscopic Gastric Bypass Surgery:

Laparoscopic Roux-en-Y Gastric Bypass was first originated by a group of Bariatric surgeons in California in 1994. This procedure is considered a combination procedure. It works by both restricting the amount of food consumed and also by providing some malabsorption. The surgical outcomes of this procedure seem to indicate that the weight loss results are similar to the traditional "open" procedure as long as the procedures are performed the same way.

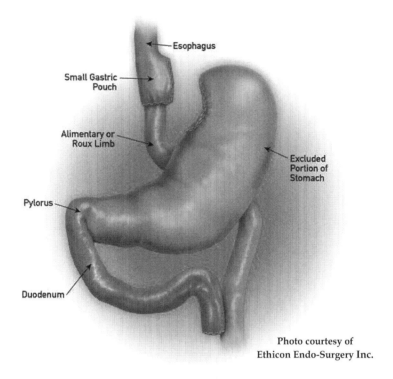

Photo courtesy of
Ethicon Endo-Surgery Inc.

The procedure begins by dividing the stomach to create a "pouch" that limits the amount of food that can be eaten. The pouch is about the size of one's thumb and can hold about 20cc or 2-3 tablespoons of food. The larger excluded stomach, known as the gastric remnant, is stapled closed and separated from the pouch. This portion no longer receives food but has a normal blood supply thereby keeping it healthy.

The second step of the procedure involves taking a portion of the small intestine and creating a "bypass" or "Roux" limb that is connected to the new pouch to provide an outlet for food. This part of the procedure is what creates a slight malabsorption of nutrients to assist in weight loss.

The malabsorptive portion of the procedure also contributes to weight loss by causing a condition known as "Dumping Syndrome". Most sugar consumed is normally absorbed in the first 1-2 feet of small intestine in normal situations. After the Gastric Bypass procedure sugar passes directly from the pouch into the lower small intestine. The unabsorbed sugar pulls fluid into the small intestine resulting in distension, increased motility (activity), cramping and a neurologic response that may cause an increase in heart rate, sweating, diarrhea, nausea, and even vomiting. Most patients will experience this at least once and will learn to avoid foods containing high sugar content, thus improving the chance for long-term weight loss success.

Risks:

- Possible conversion to an open procedure due to limited access and visibility

- There may be an increased risk for bowel obstruction in the long term

- Death (1:500-1,000)

- Pouch leaks – (1%)

- Deep venous thrombosis (1-2%)

- Pulmonary emboli (1%)

- Abdominal wall hernia (1%)

- Peptic ulcer disease (3-5%)

- Stricture (narrowing) at gastric pouch (1-2%)

- Small bowel obstruction (1-2%)

Typical Results and Outcomes:

The average best weight loss for this procedure is 70% of a individual's body weight (i.e. if someone is 100 lbs. over their ideal body weight, average weight loss outcomes would be 70 lbs.).

A weight loss of only about 40% of excess body weight will often show significant improvement in many other medical problems:

- Many Type 2 diabetics will get off of their medications

- Hypertensive clients will have improvement or resolution of their hypertension

- Sleep apnea almost always improves

- Cholesterol improvement in most clients

- Arthritic symptoms improve

Determining which procedure is right for you will require an evaluation with your surgeon and discussion about your specific situation. As you meet with him/her you will want to find out what their opinion is regarding the preferred weight loss procedure based upon your medical history as well as the number of procedures he/she has performed and their individual outcomes.

Rhonda's Opinion: *The decision has to be yours, but I am REALLY happy with the sleeve gastrectomy!*

CHAPTER 2

How Do I Know If I Qualify
for Weight Loss Surgery?

If you are at least 50 pounds over your ideal body weight and have been unsuccessful with other methods of weight loss, you may be a candidate for weight loss surgery. However, most insurance companies additionally require a BMI of 40 or greater or a BMI of 35-40 with other potentially life threatening health problems such as diabetes, high blood pressure and/or sleep apnea.

Your BMI is your weight in relation to your height. So how do you calculate your BMI? You need to take your weight in kilograms and divide by the square of your height (meters). For example, If your weight is 80 kilograms and your height is 1.8 meters, you would square your height (1.82=3.24) and then divide it into your weight (80 divided by 3.24 = a BMI of 24.69). Or you can simply enter your information online for quick results with a BMI calculator.[3]

General BMI classification guidelines include:

BMI	Classification	Health Risk
Under 18.5	Underweight	Minimal
18.5-24.9	Normal Weight	Minimal
25-29.9	Overweight	Increased
30-34.9	Obese	High
35-39.9	Severely Obese	Very High
40 and Over	Morbidly Obese	Extremely High

The decision as to whether or not weight loss surgery is right for you is ideally made by you and your surgeon after careful consideration of your weight, your past medical/surgical history and your current health problems or co-morbidities. However, there are general guidelines that most surgeons and insurance companies adhere to when choosing who an appropriate candidate for weight loss surgery is as noted below:

General Guidelines for Weight Loss Surgery Candidates:[4]

- BMI of 40 or greater

- Co-morbidity: You have a life-shortening disease process, heart disease, diabetes or obstructive sleep apnea that can be improved by losing weight.

- For at least two years, you have attempted to lose weight.

- You have been obese for an extended period of time, at least three to five years.

- You are able to effectively care for yourself and follow a physician's instructions.

- You are motivated to lose weight and maintain a healthful lifestyle.

- You do not abuse drugs or alcohol.

- You are a nonsmoker or have quit smoking.

- You are an adult under the age of 65.

These guidelines vary by insurance carrier and your individual policy. Your insurance policy is an agreement between you and your insurance provider. However, if you are working with an experienced bariatric surgeon/center, they can easily help you navigate through your particular insurance requirements and efficiently submit your information for surgery authorization. This topic is covered further in Chapter 6.

As with any general guidelines, there are caveats that cannot be ignored. Some of the ones we find most important include age, motivation and mindset. With regards to age, you can see by the general guidelines listed previously that it is recommended that an adult be under the age of 65.

At the Center for Weight Loss Success (www.cfwls.com) we do not put a cap on age for good reason. Age is just a number. You likely know someone who is over 65 years of age yet physically, emotionally and intellectually they are really more like a 40 year old. Conversely, you likely know someone around 40 who walks, talks and acts as if they are 80+ years old. In terms of lower age restrictions, although there are a few centers in the United States performing weight loss procedures on patients under the age of 18, most surgeons prefer to wait until you are 18 years of age or older and able to better decide and commit to such a life changing procedure.

Of great importance is your motivation and mindset. If you are considering weight loss surgery, you need to be motivated and an active participant throughout your entire pre-operative and post-operative phases. This is how you will experience the best results.

Weight loss surgery is something you need to do for yourself, not someone else. You need to prepare yourself physically and mentally prior to surgery and proactively plan for your post-operative phase. If you believe surgery is a "quick fix" or the "easy way out" you likely should not pursue weight loss surgery. With this mindset, you may not fully commit to the lifestyle changes that result in the rewarding outcomes that will transform your life in so many positive ways. However, if you do commit, get ready for an amazing journey.

Don't allow the process to overwhelm you. Just take it one step at a time. An experienced bariatric surgeon/center will provide a comprehensive process to help guide you through all these considerations.

Finally, it is important to note that some people are actually too obese to qualify for weight loss surgery. If you are too heavy, you will usually be instructed to lose weight before your surgeon can proceed with weight loss surgery. Once again, an experienced bariatric surgeon/center will guide you through this process and help you optimize your physical and emotional health prior to surgery and beyond.

Rhonda's Opinion: You should qualify yourself instead of letting a stranger at an insurance company make your health decisions for you.

CHAPTER 3

How Do I Know If Weight Loss Surgery Is Right for Me?

As you have read, weight loss surgery is a decision that requires research (like you are doing here), a risk/benefit comparison, an evaluation by an experienced bariatric surgeon and soul searching on your part to make sure you are committed to long-term changes. These changes can drastically improve your health, your ability to live your life to the fullest and potentially extend your lifespan. This may seem overwhelming but the important thing for you to know is that you are not alone.

There is a delay with regards to documented statistics, but here are the clear trends:

• About 15 million adults in the U.S. have morbid obesity which is associated with more than 30 other diseases and conditions including type 2 diabetes, heart disease, sleep apnea, hypertension, asthma, cancer, joint problems and infertility. The direct and indirect costs to the health care system associated with obesity are about $117 billion annually.[5]

• In the United States, the number of people who qualify for weight loss surgery is increasing as the incidence of obesity and morbid obesity is on the rise.

• In the United States, the number of weight loss procedures performed each year continues to rise with an estimated 177,600 procedures performed in 2006 (an increase from about 16,000 in the early 1990's).5 In 2008, the number of weight loss procedures was up to 220,000 and remained there in 2009. Numbers for subsequent years have not been published as of this publication.

Telling you that you are not alone and sharing these sobering statistics doesn't solve the problem for you or the general population. There has to be a need (and clearly there is a need), there has to be a want (which usually results from the pain endured as a result of being obese or morbidly obese) and finally there has to be a viable solution (in this case, surgical weight loss with an experienced bariatric surgeon who is passionate not just about surgery but your long-term health success – see Chapter 17).

Sounds like a recipe for success but there is an ingredient that is missing. You can have a need, a want and a viable solution but if you don't have the commitment and motivation to follow through and create lasting change for yourself, you may never experience the optimal success you deserve.

If you decide that you have the want, the need and the commitment, you are a great candidate for weight loss surgery. Now you just need to explore the rest of the questions in this book and get started on your path to success.

Rhonda's Opinion: It's right when you can't stay at a healthy fitness level for your age.

Keisha's Story

I started out at 230 pounds and lost 95 pounds. I was borderline hypertensive, had severe back pain and was exhausted most of the time. It was difficult to even go up a flight of stairs without being out of breath. I realized that I had to make a choice. I did my homework and made an educated decision to stop the situation early. I realized that weight loss surgery was the answer for me. I truly believe that I was given a second chance in life. I took surgery seriously, did what I was supposed to do and went from a size 20 to size 6! I couldn't be happier. Dr. Clark gave me the opportunity to get my life back and I am forever grateful.

I believe a strong support system is really important. Having education, a support group and a surgeon who listened to me, answered all of my questions and guided me to success made all of the difference. This is a life changing situation. I made a change and I am living life to the fullest and you can too!

Keisha Before Surgery

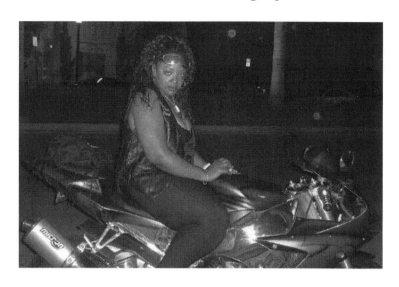

After

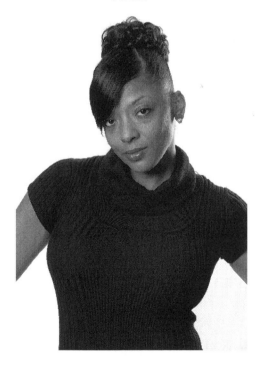

CHAPTER 4

SHOULD WEIGHT LOSS SURGERY
BE MY LAST RESORT?

You may think this is a strong statement but…ABSOLUTELY NOT! However, weight loss surgery shouldn't be your first option either. The purpose here is not to create confusion but to reinforce the fact that for people who are morbidly obese and have tried other nutritional, behavioral and fitness programs without success, weight loss surgery can be a great option.

An ideal candidate is someone who is somewhere between 75 and 150 pounds over their ideal body weight. As your weight increases, generally so does the incidence of other health problems. With the additional weight and health problems, your risk for weight loss surgery increases significantly as well. Thus, you take the risks associated with surgery and increase them which is not the most desirable situation for you or your surgeon.

The fear and negative connotations surrounding weight loss surgery has significantly decreased since 1994 when I began my weight loss surgery career. Thank goodness! In addition, the procedures have evolved and become safer and more effective. However, the higher your BMI and co-morbid conditions (other health problems) the higher your surgical risk will be. In addition, the higher the BMI and co-morbid conditions, the higher the possibility is that you may not be a candidate for weight loss surgery today.

Just because you are not an ideal candidate don't despair. Talk to your physician or a qualified bariatric surgeon in your area to find out how to reach a more optimal situation.

Rhonda's Opinion: I should have done surgery a long time ago before I yo-yoed all those years.

Tina's Story

I have successfully lost 170 lbs since my gastric sleeve surgery with Dr. Clark and the staff of the Center for Weight Loss Success. If you are considering weight loss surgery this is the place for you. The education and support that you will receive before, during, and after surgery is phenomenal! You could not ask for a better group of caring, loving individuals to care for you during a critical life-changing decision!

My journey for a healthier, confident life has not been easy. I made the decision to change the outcome of my future when I weighed an astounding 431 pounds. I was slowly killing myself. I was taking 10 to 11 pills along with insulin injections daily to keep my blood sugars under control and reduce fluid buildup around my heart. I couldn't walk a flight of stairs in my own condo. Even more I was killing my confidence that I would ever be healthy again or able to care for myself. I was only 43 years old. I was placing a fearsome burden on my 23-year-old daughter. After a hospital false alarm my family doctor told me I should consider weight loss surgery before my body began to shut down from the extra weight and that I might only have 10 more years to live. I went home and looked in the mirror at the person I had become and knew it wasn't me.

The journey began after attending the weight loss seminar at the Center for Weight Loss Success. I made the appointment, gathered all the information from the doctor and nurses. I went home read and researched once again. Then I made the phone call that changed my life forever. I scheduled my gastric sleeve surgery. I was terrified, but my fears were quickly calmed by the nurses, doctors, and staff at the Center for Weight Loss Success. They explained everything in detail, answered all my questions and my sister and daughter's questions. They gave me all the support and assistance that any person could ask for when making a life-changing decision such as this.

I followed the program, attended every nutritional counseling session, every doctor's appointment, and as many educational classes as I could. I went to group exercise classes; I worked out with my trainer and got the information I needed. There would be curve balls thrown my way from gall bladder removal surgery to the death of my mother 9 months after surgery. It was hard work, determination, and wonderful support from family, friends (especially the ones I met at CFWLS), and the Center for Weight Loss Success Staff that helped me succeed in my weight loss goals.

My journey has not ended but only begun into a new, better, healthier life for me. I have lost 170 pounds and I am still looking to loose more. The difference is I know I can do it because I have the tools, knowledge, and determination to see it through.

To the Center for Weight Loss Success staff, I will be forever indebted to you for making me see that I can reach any goal I set.

Tina Before Surgery

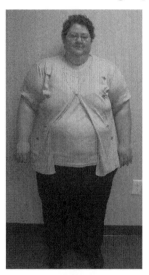

After

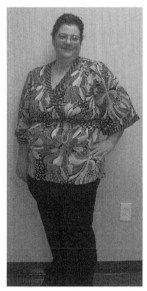

CHAPTER 5

IS WEIGHT LOSS SURGERY REVERSIBLE?

The answer is "yes" and "no" depending upon the type of weight loss surgery procedure that is performed. The bottom line is that *you should not go into weight loss surgery with the mindset that it is reversible.*

First time (primary) weight loss procedures have risk. Secondary operations have a much higher risk primarily due to potential scar tissue, potential hernia formation and the fact that your anatomy has already been altered to a certain degree depending upon the type of primary operation performed. Weight loss surgery may be reversible for the adjustable gastric banding procedure since the device can be removed. With the gastric bypass, it is anatomically reversible since the parts of the stomach and small intestine can technically be put together again, but it is not recommended and carries a higher degree of risk.

For the sleeve gastrectomy, this procedure is not reversible since the portion of the stomach that is removed in order to create your new "medium banana sized" pouch cannot be replaced.

You have to go back to your need, your desire and your motivation for surgery. It's a commitment that can reap benefits beyond your imagination. Fear is natural and you have to make sure you have done your research and you are as comfortable as possible with your decision. A certain amount of anxiety is actually desirable. It usually means that you realize you are making an important decision that will require a behavioral change (which is scary) but if you choose carefully and surround yourself with supportive people and proactively prepare for the potential obstacles, success will follow.

Rhonda's Opinion: *I don't want to ruin a great thing!*

CHAPTER 6

WILL MY INSURANCE COVER WEIGHT LOSS SURGERY?

Insurance coverage for weight loss surgery varies by state and by the insurance provider. While some insurers may cover the entire bill, many public or private insurance companies will pay a percentage (usually around 80%) of what is considered "customary and usual" for the surgery as determined by the insurance company.

The first step if you are considering weight loss surgery is to contact your insurance provider (use the provider number on your insurance card) and ask "Is weight loss surgery a covered benefit under my policy?"

Many policies require that the employer providing the policy purchase a "Ryder" for weight loss surgery. Thus, you might also want to ask "Do I have the Ryder for weight loss surgery on my policy?" The employer must purchase this Ryder for everyone that is covered under the plan, not just a select few. There are a number of factors that play into this decision for employers. However, generally speaking, employers who understand the value of weight loss and the employee benefits (improved/resolved co-morbidities, lower health care and medication costs, less time missed from work and increased productivity to name a few) are more likely to purchase the weight loss surgery Ryder.

If your initial attempt to authorize coverage is denied, you can appeal, and you should initiate your appeal immediately. Your experienced bariatric surgeon/center will assist you with this process. It makes good fiscal sense for your insurer to foot the bill for your weight loss surgery. According to the Obesity Action Coalition, the upfront costs of weight loss surgery are paid off in three and a half years, due to hospitalization cost savings.

What's more, the cost of drugs for people with diabetes and high blood pressure plummet following weight loss surgery.

Many are able to stop taking such medications altogether as their blood sugar and blood pressure return to normal levels after weight loss6.

Medicare, the U.S. government health plan as know today for people 65 years of age or older states it will pay for three types of weight loss surgery for patients who are treated in "high-volume" centers that achieve low mortality rates. The three types of surgeries as we know it today include:

- The Roux-en-Y bypass

- Open and laparoscopic biliopancreatic diversions

- Laparoscopic adjustable gastric banding

You will notice that as of this publication, the Sleeve Gastrectomy procedure is not covered by Medicare. An experienced bariatric surgeon/center can guide you through the Medicare requirements that need to be documented prior to scheduling surgery. Medicare does not pre-authorize weight loss surgery so you will need to make sure all requirements are met prior to surgery and submitted properly with your claim.

Some private insurers require a letter of medical necessity from a doctor before they will agree to pay for weight loss surgery. However, Medicare does not require pre-certification and does not pre-authorize weight loss surgery. As a result, many surgeons may ask Medicare patients to sign a contract stating that they will pay for any costs that Medicare does not cover after processing the claim. You can find out your specific requirements regarding diet history by contacting your local Medicare provider.

At the time of this publication, weight loss surgery is an option for Medicare beneficiaries if they have a body mass index (BMI) of 35, with at least one health problem related to obesity such as heart disease or diabetes. As you are aware, governmental insurance is currently under debate and potential revision. Thus, you will want to work closely with your experienced bariatric surgeon/center to address your specific situation.

Rhonda's Opinion: *It wasn't covered by my insurance – that's ok – just do it and move into the future. As I said earlier, you should qualify yourself instead of letting a stranger at an insurance company make your health decisions for you.*

Lawrence's Story

In my 40s I did a "reality check" and acknowledge that this body is not invincible. I have lost seemingly healthy friends to heart attacks, strokes, or some unexpected issue and I decided that I'm not going to let weight, poor eating habits or controllable health related concerns take me out of here!

I'm a young family and businessman; I spent my early adult years "life coaching" others on being the best them they can be, yet I neglected "me". Professionally, I was experiencing my dreams, and though I was never diagnosed with any health issues I decided to "life coach" myself because I could feel my body changing.

You can't invest in anything else until you invest in yourself. So I educated myself, challenged myself, set realistic goals and connected the dots to my purpose. Although that may sound selfish, it is actually one of the most selfless things you can do. You see I owned that I needed to be healthy, I needed to have stamina, and I needed my image to be authentically me. All roads led to Dr Clark and his wonderful team at CFWLS!

Weight loss surgery and the comprehensive program at CFWLS has been the right decision for me. I lost 101 pounds. If you are unsure about anything or have any questions, come see Dr. Clark and his team. This is the place with the answers you need and they will help you make it happen so you can exceed your goals. I have no regrets. I'm truly loving life and this journey every step of the way!

Before

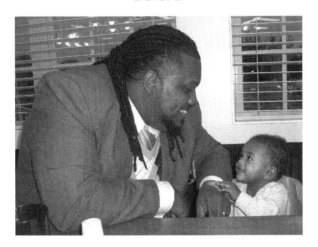

After

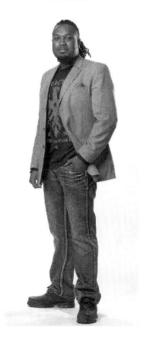

CHAPTER 7

What If My Insurance Doesn't Cover Weight Loss Surgery?

If your insurance doesn't cover weight loss surgery, you are not alone. Unfortunately, according to the American Society for Metabolic and Bariatric Surgery, less than 1 percent of those who meet the criteria for surgery actually have surgery5. A big reason for this is lack of insurance coverage.

If you find you do not have insurance coverage, there are self-pay options available (some more affordable than others). The self-pay cost of weight loss surgery procedures varies by the type of procedure and geographical area in which it is offered (urban areas tend to have a higher fee).

Generally speaking, the average cost for a gastric bypass ranges from $18,000 to $25,000, while the adjustable gastric banding surgery costs anywhere from $17,000 to $30,000. The sleeve gastrectomy procedure is newer and a price range is not as readily available. A ballpark range is anywhere from $14,000 to $22,000. The price range is also influenced by the supportive program aspects that may or may not be included, the number of follow-up visits, and for the laparoscopic adjustable banding, whether or not any adjustments are included.

The self-pay cost of weight loss surgery generally includes the cost of anesthesia, the hospital facility fee and the surgeon's fee. There may also be additional costs for diet and fitness plans, behavioral modification therapy and nutritional products before and/or after surgery. However, some fees include these services.

For example, at the Center for Weight Loss Success (www.cfwls.com), as of the time this book was published, our comprehensive weight loss surgery pricing including the costs for anesthesia, the hospital and the surgeon is as follows:

- Gastric Sleeve - $13,995.00

- Laparoscopic Adjustable Gastric Band - $16,995.00

- Gastric Bypass - $18,995

In addition, an exclusive comprehensive 12 month program is included with these fees. It is called Weight Management University for Weight Loss Surgery™ and includes the following:

Weight Management University for Weight Loss Surgery™

Pre-Operative Program:

- Comprehensive Pre-Operative Education Class

- WMU for WLS™ Curriculum Guide Book

- Access to WMU for WLS™ Recorded Webinars

- Getting Started Package - Protein Supplements

- Journal

- Shaker Cup

- CFWLS Tote Bag

- Subscription to Monthly e-Newsletter

- 10% Coupon for Nutritional Store

- CFWLS Rewards Card (credit toward future store purchases)

Post-Operative Program:

- WMU for WLS™ Modules - Including chapter, DVD & CD delivered monthly to your door

- Weekly Live Webinars with Dr. Clark

- Individualized Counseling Sessions

- Access to "Member Only" Portal

- 3-30 Minute Personal Training Sessions

- Weekly Lifestyle & Behavior Modification Class

- Unlimited Group Fitness Classes

- Unlimited Body Composition Analysis

- Monthly Support Group Meetings

- Monthly In-Store Events

You may be surprised that all of these products/services are included, but it's the right thing to do for optimal long-term results and has resulted in a high degree of patient satisfaction and improved outcomes. For those that travel for surgery, some services are offered online instead of on-site. No matter who you choose as your bariatric surgeon, make sure that there is a comprehensive program available and ongoing support prior, during and after surgery.

Also, most experienced bariatric surgeons/centers have financing options available. You will want to verify this and explore your options. How much is adding 5-7 years of quality life worth to you?

Rhonda's Opinion: You will find a way to pay for it...I did and I did not make very much money at the time at all. You are worth it and Dr. Clark's program is one of the most comprehensive and affordable programs available anywhere.

Alesha's Story

I want to say a big Thank You to Dr. Clark and his staff at the Center for Weight Loss Success (CFWLS). Being a self-pay client, I could have gone with the cheapest doctor but I really wanted to make sure I went with a surgeon that offered the keys to long-term weight loss success. Dr. Clark and the CFWLS staff are second to none. I am thankful to have at my disposal his nutritional information, products and classes; support groups, dietician, fitness center and personal trainers; as well as his insurance coordinator and supporting staff. The team is superb and so is Dr. Clark's bedside manner!

These sentiments are repeatedly confirmed when I see patients from other doctors coming to our support groups because their doctors lack the support and guidance that Dr. Clark and his staff offer. When we compare our losses (I am down a 185 pounds and still loosing) and long-term accomplishments, theirs pale in comparison to ours. I thank God for the blessing that Dr. Clark and the CFLWS team have been in my life. I could not have done it without all of them!

Before

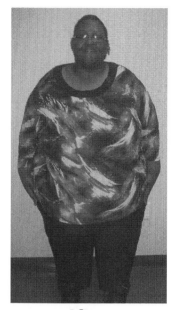

After

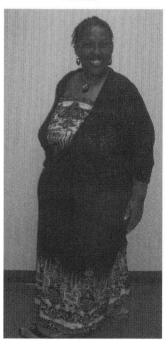

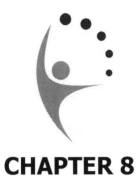

CHAPTER 8

How Can I Be Best Prepared for Weight Loss Surgery?

"By failing to prepare you are preparing to fail."

--Benjamin Franklin

How to be best prepared for weight loss surgery is one of those questions that might not be on the top of your list, but will contribute to your overall level of success. As you know, weight loss surgery is an important decision. If you are adequately prepared, your level of anxiety will decrease and you will be better able to manage the changes required of you after surgery. In addition, with preparation comes confidence. This is a great trait to have as you embark upon this remarkable journey.

So how do you prepare for weight loss surgery? You will want to ask questions. You will want to make sure that your bariatric surgeon/center has a very thorough educational process in place prior to and after surgery that addresses nutrition, behavior modification and fitness. **These three components are critical to long-term success.**

You may only be thinking short-term. Let's face it, you are really busy and have many obligations at home, at work, with school and with friends that take precedence over your needs. It's easy to tell yourself "I will figure this out" but it is a lot easier if you have a support system in place at home and with your bariatric surgeon/center prior to surgery so that you can better manage any surprises that may come along the way.

If you have already decided to have weight loss surgery, you will want to think about the positive changes you want to accomplish. Often people view surgery from a number perspective (i.e. how many pounds they would like to lose). Weight loss surgery is about so much more than that. It is about enabling yourself to accomplish things that might not have been possible in the past. It is about having an exciting life. Life you can experience to the fullest extent. It is very important to think about (and document) life goals related to your weight loss. Then you can celebrate the positive changes transforming your life.

Some of the "dreams" that people have shared include:

- Walking up the stairs or to the corner of their street without getting short of breath

- Playing with their children or grandchildren

- Crossing their legs

- Painting their toenails

- Stop worrying about being able to fit into a chair at a public place or worrying that it will break when they sit on it

- Fitting in a bathtub and having water on both sides

- Shopping in a store for regular sized people

- Riding a bicycle

- Returning to a productive lifestyle

- Stop worrying about going to a restaurant that might only have booths or chairs with arms on them

- Going to a movie and fitting into the seat

Take some time to identify your "wish list" and document it. Then spend some time getting your mind and body ready. In the weeks or days before surgery, you need to consider yourself in training. Just as athletes prepare for a race, you can prepare yourself to be in top form for surgery. When you actively get your body and mind ready you likely will:

- Have fewer complications from anesthesia and surgery

- Be able to cooperate with necessary treatments

- Heal faster and feel better quicker

- Have better control of your pain

There are some very specific things you need to do to be in the best shape possible. You need to begin these things as soon as possible. We know that the very worst time to try to learn things is right after surgery when you may feel foggy from anesthesia and uncomfortable from your operation. Learn and practice these things now so that you will be able to help yourself after surgery.

- **Focus on healthy eating.** The better nourished you are, the more quickly your tissues will heal. Healing is WORK for your body. Good nutrition helps you tolerate the stresses on your body and to offset limits on food and fluids right after surgery. Weight loss prior to your surgery can decrease your risk and improve recovery time after surgery. This is why you should incorporate your new eating plan and individualized weight loss counseling prior to surgery as a part of your overall plan. Consult your bariatric surgeon for specific options for weight loss prior to surgery.

- **If you are a smoker – QUIT!** Even a few weeks of not smoking increases the safety of anesthesia. You will not be allowed to smoke while hospitalized. You will need all your oxygen for healing.

- **Build your exercise tolerance.** Toning your muscles and building your strength will help you bounce back quicker. Walking is a perfect exercise for you prior to surgery. It is normal to feel a little weak after surgery, but you can reduce this by toning up with daily exercise.

- **Exercise your lungs!** Practice your deep breathing. After surgery you will be encouraged to do this. Expanding your lungs helps your system get rid of anesthesia drugs quickly, helps prevent pneumonia, and speeds oxygen to your tissues to help you heal quickly. You will also FEEL better.

- **Move your legs to prevent blood clots!!!!** After an operation, the best exercise to help your circulation and reduce your chance of blood clots will be walking! The nurses in the hospital will get you up after a brief recovery period following surgery. Once you go home, follow the specific discharge instructions set forth by your surgeon. In general, you should rest as needed but also get up and walk around as much as you can tolerate. You can do these exercises in bed or sitting in a chair during any rest periods.

○ Lying on your back in bed, "walk" your feet toward your body until your knees are fully bent. Tighten your abdominal muscles while you do this. Now let your legs slide gently back to the flat position and repeat this four more times.

○ Lying in bed or sitting up, point your toes as if you were trying to bend your foot backwards. Hold for the count of five and relax. You should feel a "pull" on the muscles in the front of your legs. Next point your heels away from your body, tightening your leg muscles. Hold for the count of five and relax. You should feel this pull in the back of your legs. Repeat the pointing exercises 5-10 times.

If you have decided to have surgery, you also need to **focus your mind on a good outcome.** You are the most important player in this team effort, and much will depend on your ability to fully participate. Your feelings and thoughts will play a very big part in your recovery. Reassure yourself that the best people, equipment and techniques are supporting you during surgery.

Finally, if you have decided to have surgery, a good way to prepare is to use the power of your relationships to gather a support group. Enlist family and friends to help you keep your spirits up. Let friends and neighbors help with chores and meals.

We all do better when we know we are supported by people who care about us and are cheering us on. Don't underestimate the power of your emotions. Positive thinking is the biggest help you can give yourself. Think hopeful, optimistic thoughts about the experience ahead, and start NOW!

If you do all of these things, you will be best prepared for a positive experience and outcome.

Rhonda's Opinion: *Do what the doctor says!*

CHAPTER 9

How Much Weight Can I Expect to Lose After Weight Loss Surgery?

Weight loss varies depending upon the surgical procedure, your pre-operative weight and your commitment to following the diet/exercise recommendations after surgery. On an average, people lose approximately 70% of what they were overweight. For example, if you were 100 pounds over your ideal body weight, you would lose an average of 70 pounds – if you were 200 pounds over your ideal body weight, you would lose an average of 140 pounds.

Prior to selecting your surgeon/bariatric center, ask them what the average weight loss is for their clients after surgery. At the Center for Weight Loss Success, the *average* weight loss after weight loss surgery is 127 pounds. That takes into account weight loss for patients who began with a BMI anywhere between 33 and 50+.

Optimal weight loss results can be attained if you do the following:

• Attend your scheduled surgeon appointments before and after surgery.

• Attend monthly support group meetings usually provided through your surgeon's office.

• Strictly follow the diet set forth by your surgeon and if he/she has made nutritional coaching and/or personal training visits available to you through their weight loss surgery program, participate fully and attend these sessions.

• Include your support person(s) in your appointments/classes/support group as appropriate so they fully understand what you need to be doing and how to support you for optimal success.

• Monitor not only your weight but your full body composition (hopefully a service provided at your weight loss surgeon's office) as you progress post-operatively. You will want to make sure you are losing fat and not your lean body mass (muscle).

• Be sure to get in enough quality protein (check with your surgeon but usually at least 90 grams per day). This will help with your overall ability to maintain your lean body mass (muscle) which drives your metabolism. It is also important for healing and prevention of potential long-term problems such as hair loss.

• Incorporate fitness as soon as your surgeon indicates it is safe for you to do so. Walking is a great beginning routine but you will want to incorporate increased cardio training and resistance training with weights. Your surgeon will likely either provide these services or provide you with an appropriate plan/resource.

• Immediately after surgery your surgeon will likely be most concerned that you are staying hydrated. Water is very important so be sure to sip all day long and in the long run get approximately 64 ounces of water in every day. In addition to proper hydration, you need to make sure you are ingesting appropriate amounts of protein as mentioned earlier.

- Take your vitamins as recommended by your surgeon and make sure they are pharmaceutical grade for optimal quality.

- Whenever you are trying to lose weight, you can improve your rate of success by journaling what you eat and drink. This also helps as you meet with your surgeon and/or the nutritional coach before and after surgery.

- Surround yourself with positive people who support your decision to have weight loss surgery.

Rhonda's Opinion: *As much as you want to and are committed to lose.*

Cyndie's Story

My life before weight loss surgery consisted of sleeping with a CPAP machine at the highest setting at night, using oxygen as needed during the day, high blood pressure, osteoporosis and COPD. I have 3 children and a husband and I was told by my doctor that if I didn't have the surgery I was going to die.

I was out of work and filing for disability. If I sat down, I would fall asleep immediately and yet when I stood up, my legs and feet swelled and hurt terribly. I could hardly walk. In fact, I was in and out of the hospital frequently for breathing problems. This was not the life I wanted to live.

I talked to others who had weight loss surgery and did my own research. I learned about Dr. Clark and his success and decided to give it a shot. I learned what I needed to know from Dr. Clark and he helped me to save my own life. Dr. Clark gave me the tool I needed to lose weight. Being overweight runs in my family. In fact, my father, mother and brother have all had weight loss surgery with Dr. Clark. Between the four of us, **we have lost over 700 pounds!** It's an amazing journey that I am glad I took it. Life is so much better and I am forever grateful for what Dr. Clark and his team have helped me to do.

Before

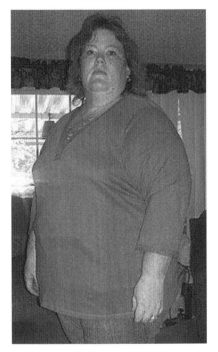

After

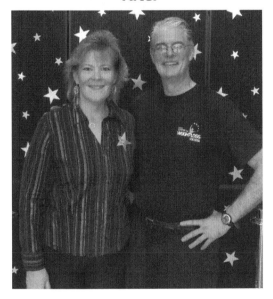

CHAPTER 10

WHAT IS LIFE LIKE AFTER WEIGHT LOSS SURGERY?

Your feelings regarding life after surgery will likely vary depending upon how far out you are from surgery, your level of preparation prior to surgery, your ability to manage change and your overall attitude/mindset. Rest assured, there is often not a dry eye in the office as goals are met/exceeded throughout the first year after surgery and beyond. It's extremely rewarding for you and everyone involved and you hear more often than not *"I wish I would have done this sooner"*.

As a generalization, at the Center for Weight Loss Success, we have found that most people go through a few expected phases and the timeframe for each varies:

Phase 1: What have I done?

Phase 2: I can do this.

Phase 3: I am glad I did this.

Phase 4: I wish I would have done this sooner!

Phase 5: I need to stay on track (especially if necessary long-term success habits throughout the first year after surgery weren't developed).

At the time of this publication, the primary surgery performed by Dr. Clark at the Center for Weight Loss Success is the sleeve gastrectomy. In fact, most of these patients go home the same day of surgery since you generally recover better in your own home environment. You go through a thorough pre-operative program and your post-operative program begins right away.

When you first go home from the hospital, here are some general guidelines for what to expect. Of course, each surgeon has their own particular orders so be sure to follow whatever he/she recommends.

- With regards to your diet, you will want to make sure you are staying hydrated by sipping all day. You will usually continue with a liquid diet until you are seen by your surgeon 10-14 days after surgery. You should not have any carbonated beverages – refer to your the liquid diet instructions set forth by your surgeon. You need to stay hydrated and do your best to try to get about 80-100 grams of protein in per day with high quality protein shakes (again, follow your surgeons specific orders).

- You will want to be up and walking as tolerated and rest when you are tired. You are usually permitted to shower. Common sense comes into play here. If anything is hurting you then you probably should not be doing it yet. At the Center for Weight Loss Success, we restrict lifting to no more than 20 pounds for the first two weeks and restrict driving for 3-4 days after surgery as long as you are off of your pain medication. Getting up and moving is a good thing. Not only for your body but for your emotional state as well.

- Your surgeon will have specific instructions for wound care and medications. Follow these as instructed.

- It is not unusual for you to question "What did I do?" the first days after surgery. It is a big adjustment and although you won't likely feel hungry, just drinking liquids is a big change and can be difficult to get used to. The first few days tend to be the worst and then you get used to it. It helps to focus on your goals. This will all be worth it.

- Make sure you go to all of your scheduled follow-up appointments and call your surgeon if you have any questions/concerns.

After the first two weeks, you will generally be able to begin "mushy" foods. At the Center for Weight Loss Success, we have a thorough educational program that guides you through exactly what to do or eat which is beyond the scope of this book. Your experienced bariatric surgeon/center will likely have similar resources for you.

At approximately one month after surgery, you will begin eating more regular foods. You will want to focus on getting in an adequate amount of quality protein (at least 90 grams), staying hydrated (sometimes thirst is mistaken for hunger) and easing into a regular exercise regimen. Your experienced bariatric surgeon/center will have an entire plan set to help guide you through each phase after surgery. Remember, it is never too early to begin your habits for success.

As a general rule, these include:

• **Eating** - Don't skip meals. Food choices should be low fat and low sugar. Think "Protein First". Eating should be approached as "how little can I eat and be satisfied", NOT "how much can I fit into my new smaller stomach". You will want to cut your food up into small pieces, use a smaller plate, put your fork/spoon down in between bites and chew slowly. It is best to eat at a table and not "on the run" so you will avoid eating too fast, overfilling your pouch and end up with unnecessary pain or difficulty.

• **Drinking** – Try to avoid drinking with your meals since it "washes" the food through quicker and decreases your ability to stay fuller longer. Beverages should be non-caloric and non-carbonated. Drinking 8 glasses of water each day is a good idea with any weight loss plan. Avoid alcoholic beverages.

• **Vitamins** – Multivitamins should be taken daily – *Forever.* Other vitamins and/or supplements may be needed depending upon individual needs.

• **Sleeping** – Make sure you are well rested. You will be most successful if you sleep an average of 7 hours each night.

• **Exercise** – Regular exercise is *extremely* important and should be done at least 3-4 times per week for *at least* 30-40 minutes.

- **Personal Responsibility** – Successful patients take personal responsibility for weight loss/weight control. *It's up to you!!* No one else can lose the weight for you. The surgery is only a "tool". You have to use this tool appropriately.

Every person recovers at a different rate. It is important to take it one day, one week, and one month at a time. Be involved in your pre-operative and post-operative educational program and try to attend a support group once a month. Being around others who are experiencing the same thing or who have a long-term success story to share is very helpful. When you get to that point, be sure to share your success as well.

Celebrate your accomplishments along the way and reward yourself with something non-food related such as a massage, manicure, pedicure, golf club, fitness center membership, new piece of exercise equipment or a great piece of clothing. You will not want to invest a large amount of money in clothing because of rapid weight loss. Joining a clothing exchange with other weight loss surgery patients is helpful too.

Finally, surround yourself with like-minded successful people who support you and your goals. There are plenty of saboteurs in this world – they may even be your closest family or friends. This is a topic we could write an entire book about! In short, ask them for their support and explain the changes you want and need to make (use "I" statements and own your goals). If they continue to be unsupportive, you may need to limit your time with them. I know this is easier said than done but it is ok for you to be selfish – this is your time to shine! Don't allow others to steal your future. Go for it!

Rhonda's Opinion: *Fantastic – I don't have my old life back – I have a better life.*

Cindy's Story

Before surgery, I had multiple health problems such as diabetes, hypertension, asthma, sleep apnea, hypothyroidism. Also, I was on multiple medications for many years. This prevented me from working for a period of time and then after I went to work, once I arrived back home, I was too tired to cook or do anything with my kids. I needed to rest.

Prior to attending a weight loss seminar with Dr. Clark, I was not set on surgery. However, after attending, I knew this was what I needed and the support has been outstanding. Since my surgery, I have lost 120 pounds and all of my health problems are reversed. I get out and I'm at the gym 4-5 nights a week and can do anything with my kids. The support has been outstanding and I am grateful.

I got my gift of health back from Dr. Clark and his staff. I am grateful. In addition, I can call anytime with questions about surgery, nutrition, fitness and/or behavior and I even volunteer at the office – it's so much fun. I'd love to help anyone contemplating surgery. It is worth it and I couldn't be happier…or more active!

Before

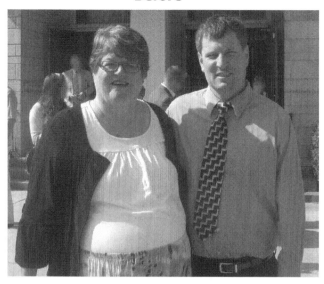

After

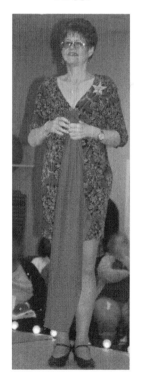

CHAPTER 11

WHY IS PROTEIN SO IMPORTANT
AFTER SURGERY?

Protein is essential with any weight loss plan. Protein is essential for muscle and tissue growth and repair. If you reduce your caloric intake without consuming the necessary amount of protein, your weight loss will be a combination of lean body mass and fat loss. With adequate protein intake (and exercise), you should be able to preserve your muscle mass, allowing the majority of your weight loss to come from fat stores. If, over time, you do not meet your daily protein needs, you may experience fatigue, loss of lean body mass, and possible hair loss.

You will need to check with your surgeon, but we recommend that our patients take in **at least 90-100 grams of protein every day.** As your weight loss continues, your body will still prefer using your lean muscle as a source of energy. Therefore, consuming 90-100 grams of protein daily will be a goal throughout your weight loss journey, not just during the beginning phases.

Once your weight has stabilized and you are in a maintenance phase then protein requirements may decrease somewhat into the 60-90 range depending on your weight and overall muscle mass. The higher your weight the more protein you may require in order to maintain Lean Body Mass. Men typically require more protein due to their higher total Lean Body Mass.

People seeking medical or surgical weight loss often have many questions surrounding protein intake since it is important for both situations. How many kinds of protein are there? Where can I find it? How much do I need? What is the best time to have it? Let's try to give some straight forward answers to these questions.

The word protein is derived from the Greek word proteios, meaning "of the first quality". Protein is essential for life (i.e. we CANNOT survive without it!!!) because it contains sulfur and nitrogen, two vital elements for every cell in your body. Protein also helps produce enzymes and hormones, maintain fluid balance, and regulate numerous vital functions, from building antibodies to building muscle. The body maintains roughly 50,000 different protein containing compounds, forming the building blocks of muscle, bone, cartilage, skin, hair and blood.

As far at your diet is concerned, there are numerous kinds of proteins, each with their own set of advantages. The right kinds can make all the difference, especially if you are trying to lose weight and build muscle. Some of the best protein comes from food. Meat has about 7 grams of protein/oz., large eggs about 7 grams of protein, and milk about 8 grams of protein/oz. In a weight loss plan, you have to watch all the extra calories (fat, carbs) that come with food sources of protein.

• **Whey Protein:** Whey protein is derived from milk (remember Little Miss Muffet and her curds and whey?). Many whey protein supplements have had most of the excess fat, cholesterol and lactose removed. Whey proteins are undoubtedly the most commonly used and most popular protein used in sports nutrition and with good reason. They are the highest quality protein available with an excellent balance of essential amino acids. Whey proteins are very efficiently absorbed and this is extremely important but this is also a potential problem. Because whey protein is so efficiently absorbed (i.e. absorbed quickly) it tends to not keep you feeling full or satisfied for any extended period of time. For this reason, it also tends to work better if used in small doses (10-20 gms) taken multiple times throughout the day. Your hunger can potentially return faster than with other proteins. This brings us to Casein protein.

• **Casein Protein:** Casein protein is also derived from milk (the curds part of curds and whey) and is essentially whey's counterpart. It also is a very high quality protein with all the essential amino acids. While whey is absorbed very rapidly, casein forms a slow digesting gel in your stomach. This in turn promotes a feeling of fullness that can stave off hunger for longer periods of time. This steady stream of amino acids helps to protect against muscle breakdown. A good casein based protein supplement made specifically for weight loss is Weight and Inches (29gm protein/serving) which can be obtained from CFWLS.

• **Egg Proteins:** Egg proteins digest at a moderate pace. Eggs are an excellent protein source and mimic the amino acid profile of muscle quite nicely. Unfortunately, eggs do have a relatively high amount of cholesterol and also arachodonic acid (mainly in the yolks). Some people are very sensitive to arachodonic acid worsening inflammatory processes. Egg proteins in supplement form (usually as albumin) have had most of the cholesterol and arachodonic acid removed.

- **Soy Protein:** Soy protein is also digested at a moderate pace. Soy protein contains all of the essential amino acids, but since soy is a plant, it tends to not have quite as good of a ratio of essential amino acids as dairy or egg based protein. Therefore, it does not tend to protect muscle mass quite as well. It can still be a good alternative for those who do not tolerate dairy based proteins.

As far as timing goes, ideally you should use smaller doses of protein multiple times throughout the day. This is especially important after weight loss surgery so even these recommendations will need to be altered somewhat during the phase immediately following surgery. Starting the day off with a good dose is always a good idea (i.e. that protein shake in the morning). An example would be 20-30 grams at breakfast, 20-30 grams at lunch and 20-30 grams at dinner. Then add two 10-20 gram snacks, appropriately spaced between meals. Positioning a protein snack prior to and immediately after strenuous exercise works extremely well to build/preserve muscle mass.

After surgery, your new stomach pouch will initially only be able to hold about 1-2 tablespoons (15-30cc) of fluid at a time. This is approximately ½-1 medicine cup. Your new stomach should eventually stretch to accommodate 6-8 ounces (3/4 to 1 cup) within the first 1-2 years after surgery. Because your new stomach pouch is so small, you need to follow the guidelines provided by your surgeon to ensure the fluid/food you put in your stomach is the most nutritious possible and does not overfill your small stomach, causing you pain and/or nausea/vomiting.

Rhonda's Opinion: *For me – anything in moderation.*

CHAPTER 12

WILL I EVER BE ABLE TO ENJOY MY FAVORITE FOODS AGAIN AFTER WEIGHT LOSS SURGERY?

Life after weight loss surgery is not all about deprivation. In fact, life after surgery is quite the contrary. It's about having an extra reinforcement so that you are better equipped to lose weight and keep it off long-term. As we have said over and over, surgery is a tool but you really need to know how best to use this tool for optimal long-term results. Our society is focused on the here and now. You will have an excellent tool that will help you quickly in the here and now after surgery. More importantly it will serve you well for the long haul so you can fully experience your life in a rewarding and active way. My team and I see dreams come true each and every day!

Sure, there will be changes and I would be lying if I said they were all going to be simple. I am not trying to be vague here but the answer to the question "Will I ever be able to enjoy my favorite foods again after weight loss surgery?" depends upon a number of things. These include the type of surgery you have and what is included in your favorite food list. Not knowing exactly what those favorite foods are, I will include those that you will need to avoid altogether or enjoy in small quantities (I always like to focus on what you *can* have rather than what you *can't* have).

The first category you will want to avoid or enjoy in small quantities is sugary sweets. This can be in solid (i.e. candy) or liquid form (i.e. sweet tea). After weight loss surgery, you should avoid food with >8 grams of sugar (5 grams if you are diabetic) because they can cause a negative reaction in your system, particularly if you have had a gastric bypass. These foods can cause what is commonly called "dumping syndrome". Dumping syndrome occurs when there is a rapid passage of food into the small intestines causing a shift of fluid to the small intestine. This usually occurs when you ingest foods that are too high in sugar or fat. Symptoms include diarrhea, sweating, nausea, cold/clammy skin, dizziness, weakness, flushed appearance, and occasionally headaches. You will need to stop and rest until the symptoms subside. Remember to remain hydrated (water is best). Take note of the food/foods that caused these symptoms so that you can avoid them in the future.

The second category you will want to avoid is alcohol. Alcohol is full of empty calories, dehydrates the body, and has negative effects on the kidneys and liver. In addition, because of the small size of your new pouch and the fact that food/liquid now empties more rapidly into the intestines, alcohol will be more toxic and cause a higher blood alcohol level than before surgery. For these reasons, ingestion of alcohol should be avoided after surgery. If you choose to have weight loss surgery and then ingest alcohol, please be aware that a small amount can affect you to a MUCH greater degree than prior to surgery.

After you are a month or so out from surgery, you can begin to experiment more with various foods. Introduce raw fruits and vegetables cautiously. Although many people do just fine, certain foods may be difficult to tolerate because your digestive system cannot handle them. The following may cause problems for you and may need to be avoided:

- Tough meats, especially hamburger. Even after grinding, the gristle in hamburger is hard to digest.

- Membranes of oranges or grapefruit

- Cores, seeds, or skins of fruits or vegetables

- Fibrous vegetables such as corn and celery

- Hulls, popcorn

- Breads - Fresh breads "ball up" in your stomach and can block your pouch. Try to avoid breads/crackers/cereals as much as possible.

- Fried foods

- Milk – If you are lactose intolerant you may use "Lactaid" products or soybean milk

- Rice – tends to expand further once in your stomach and can cause pain

This list may seem daunting but realize that the further you are out from surgery, the more tolerant your system tends to be. However, it is very important that especially throughout the first year you participate in a comprehensive program which should be available with any experienced bariatric surgeon/center. A comprehensive program should include:

- Follow-up visits with your surgeon.

- Individualized coaching with a nutrition specialist who

understands the needs of the weight loss surgery patient.

- Personal trainer/fitness center that eases you into appropriate exercise activities in a safe and comfortable environment.

- Access to delicious nutritional products that support your need for 90+ grams of protein each day.

- An ongoing support group for you and your family/significant others.

All of this is provided on-site or online at the Center for Weight Loss Success and truly impacts the short and long-term outcomes of our awesome patients. For those that live farther away, most services are very effectively provided online, via Skype, via webinars and other engaging ways. Short and long-term comprehensive support is essential for optimal success.

Rhonda's Opinion: Absolutely! I enjoy food in moderation even more than before because it tastes so much better when you slow down to enjoy it.

Ken's Story

I used to have a pharmacy on my microwave for all of the medications I had to take for diabetes, high blood pressure and high cholesterol. One day, I went in for a routine check-up and at the same time I am telling my doctor I have to do something, he handed me a brochure for Dr. Clark. I knew I had to do something and for me, weight loss surgery was the answer.

Now that am on the other side…I can honestly say it's a challenge at times. I still get excited about foods I love and have to remind myself to slow down. With all of the education from Dr. Clark and the staff at CFWLS, my choices are so much better. In fact, I probably read more labels than books these days!

I have done all of the diets, diet pills and even hypnosis in the past. I realize that this is the last "diet" I will ever have to go on. Every step is an education but it is a journey worth taking. This surgery has helped me break old habits and is the only thing that has been successful.

I truly feel like the reset button has been pushed and I am back in my 20's again in terms of how I feel and my overall energy level. I walked on the treadmill 1.5 miles at the gym last night without even breaking a sweat. I used to huff and puff just going a very short distance though. I am stronger and regaining lost life.

We all have to make the decision that is right for us. I highly recommend weight loss surgery and recommend that you listen and follow everything they tell you to do before, during and after. Dr. Clark has thankfully helped me save my life!

Before

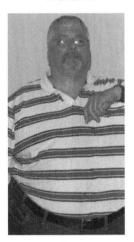

After

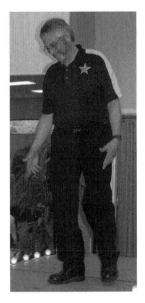

CHAPTER 13

HOW SOON CAN I GO BACK TO WORK AFTER WEIGHT LOSS SURGERY?

This decision regarding your ability to return to work will need to be made by your surgeon. He/she is best equipped to determine your return to work date since they know what procedure you had, any other health problems that you have and your recovery status.

However, in general, after a minimally invasive procedure without any complications, you will be able to return to work (with lifting restrictions for 2 weeks) within 1 week after surgery.

I recommend you take 2 weeks off after surgery so that you can adjust to your initial liquid diet in your own environment but I certainly have had people go back to work much sooner without difficulty. Once again, it goes back to your level of preparedness, your motivation, your healing and your mental attitude.

Rhonda's Opinion: *Soon – but it is dependent upon what you do for a living – be sure to check with your surgeon.*

CHAPTER 14

What If I Lose Too Much Weight?

You wouldn't think this would be a commonly asked question but it is. You may have heard a horror story about a "person who had weight loss surgery and lost so much weight that they look pale, weak and all of their skin sags". This is by far the exception and not the norm.

Weight loss after weight loss surgery is consistent and rapid (primarily with the gastric bypass and sleeve gastrectomy procedures and not as rapid with the laparoscopic adjustable gastric banding procedure). Eventually, the body recognizes this rapid weight loss and as a protective mechanism, will slow down your metabolism and you will experience a plateau. By following your prescribed eating plan (we make it as simple as possible) and incorporating fitness, you can work through these plateaus.

Once you get closer to your goal weight, the body naturally stabilizes at an appropriate weight even if you continue with a lower food intake (if it is the right combination of macronutrients and overall calories). The industry commonly calls this the "set point". If you did continue to lose weight and appear as if you were dropping below your ideal body weight (rare), we can teach you how to use your "tool" to gain weight as well.

If you looked like the person described previously, you would need to be sure you were following up with your experienced bariatric surgeon. Some things that can contribute to such a situation include poor nutrition, lack of an adequate amount of protein, not taking your daily vitamin, iron deficiency, smoking, depression or a physical malabsorption problem. Again, this is a rare situation. If you follow the prescribed post-operative comprehensive program set forth by your experienced bariatric surgeon/center this would be avoided.

Rhonda's Opinion: I actually did lose a little too much weight but worked with Dr. Clark and a trainer to gain back muscle. The great thing is that now YOU have CONTROL!!!

Wanda's Story

In 2006, I saw my dad lying in the hospital after having a pace maker put in for his heart. I inherited his family genes of being overweight, high blood pressure, high cholesterol and I saw myself in that bed. Right then I decided I was going to have gastric bypass surgery.

I had my surgery and it was a breeze. By the time I went in for my first check-up, I had lost 35 pounds in just 2-3 weeks. I have been overweight all my life and my heaviest weight was 325 pounds. I could not run or walk long distances. I had to have a knee replacement due to all the weight I had been carrying.

After surgery when I started to plateau and maintain, I had lost a total of 185 pounds. A little too much in my opinion, but with the help of Dr. Clark and his wonderful office staff I was able to maintain my weight loss and then actually put on some weight to get to a better size for me. It has been over 7 years since my weight loss surgery and I have maintained 120-130 pounds of lost weight. I wish I had done this year's ago!

I have grandkids now and I am very active. I can run, climb on the playground equipment and get down on the floor and play with them. I also go fishing with my husband and dance. I cannot even list all the things I can do now after the weight loss. I feel better and no longer need to take any of my high blood pressure medicines or cholesterol medicines (notice this is plural since I was on numerous medications).

Now I take vitamins, drink plenty of water, exercise as much as I can. I can even walk circles around my grandkids sometimes. I would recommend this to anybody who is considering having surgery. Dr. Clark and his office staff are always there to help you and answer any questions you have. They are never in a hurry and treat you like family. Even now, over 7 years out from my surgery, if I hit a bump in the road all I have to do is call and they are right there to help me get back on track.

Before

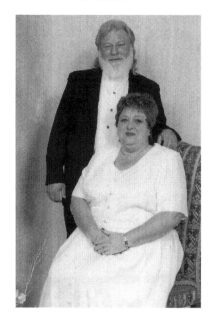

After

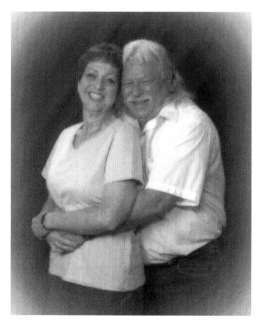

CHAPTER 15

WILL I HAVE TO EXERCISE AFTER WEIGHT LOSS SURGERY?

The short answer is "Yes". Exercise is extremely important following weight loss surgery because you will be losing weight at a rapid pace. Your body will try to fight this weight loss by attempting to store fat for this perceived starvation. Your body does this by burning muscle mass and storing fat. This is undesirable. To combat this effect, it is important to exercise regularly so that your metabolism is increased and your body burns fat rather than muscle mass.

If you decide to have weight loss surgery, you should seize this opportunity before and after surgery by integrating activity/exercise into your daily routine. This will not only help you through any plateaus, it will help you build muscle, enhance your metabolism and overall energy, and greatly influence your overall success.

I encourage walking beginning the day of surgery to improve circulation. Early walking forces the heart to pump blood throughout the body and prevents it from pooling in your legs which could cause clots that are potentially life threatening. The more walking you can do, the better. We ask that you avoid lifting heavy weights or doing sit-ups/abdominal crunches until you are at least 4 weeks from your surgery. Prior to that time, you may ride an exercise bike, or swim (but not until 2 weeks from your surgery). When you choose your particular exercise program, make sure it incorporates weight training along with some form of aerobic/cardiovascular exercise.

Most everyone knows the benefits of exercise – it's just doing it that is difficult. We all can find excuses (not enough time, not enjoyable/boring, inconvenient, lack of resources, don't know how, etc…). The bottom line is that you must **make time for exercise and make it a priority.** This is easy to say, but hard to do.

The benefits of exercise are many. Some of these benefits include:

- Decreased appetite

- Decreased blood pressure

- Decreased stress level

- Reduced risk for development of heart disease

- Reduced risk for colon and other cancers

- Reduced depression and anxiety

- Improved balance and independent living

- Improved digestion

- Improved self-esteem

- Improved flexibility

- Improved energy levels

- Improved sleep pattern

- Improved sexual satisfaction

- Improved overall quality of life

So you may logically understand the benefits of exercise. If you still choose not to exercise, you must ask yourself "why?" Determine your roadblocks to exercise and then identify solutions to the roadblock. Once you "get the fever" for exercise after doing some form on a regular basis, you will wonder why you didn't do it earlier. If you choose weight loss surgery, you are making a life changing decision.

Maximize the benefits of this decision and commit to a regular exercise program. You will not regret it. Your weight loss will be enhanced and your overall quality of life improved.

It does take time and effort to get started. In addition, after you have had surgery, you may have some feelings of fatigue for the first one to three months after surgery. Until you can begin a more vigorous exercise program (4 weeks after surgery), walk as much as possible. If you are unable to walk due to a health problem/disability, perform as much upper body exercise as you can tolerate using light weights (until 4 weeks after surgery). If you have cardiac/respiratory problems, be sure to obtain clearance for starting an exercise program from your primary care physician and/or specialist.

Choose a fitness program that will work for you. It should be tailored to your specific needs, abilities, preferences and activities that you will enjoy. Otherwise, you will be tempted to quit.

Remember that at the Center for Weight Loss Success, we love making fitness fun and specialize in starting wherever you are. We work privately with our patients and offer three personal training sessions as a part of their Weight Management University for Weight Loss Surgery™ program. Our certified trainers love working with clients at all levels of fitness. You can also participate in our Group Fitness classes as a part of your program. Remember, you are not alone. Please use these resources available with your experienced bariatric surgeon/center to enhance your weight loss and improve your overall health and metabolism.

When starting a workout program, take it easy. Be sure to gradually work up to at least 30 minutes of vigorous exercise three or more times a week. Stick to it and strive to make exercise a habit (usually considered a habit once performed regularly for at least three months)! You won't see dramatic changes overnight but you will see dramatic changes over time.

When you exercise, be sure to warm-up prior to the activity and cool down/stretch after the activity. Do not lift too much weight (increase weight gradually), and remain hydrated – be sure to drink water before and after your workout.

Rhonda's Opinion: *You will want to move because you will feel better with the weight off! This will feed your desire to become active because you hurt less and less until one day you feel great!*

Tony's Story

My name is Tony. I live in Yorktown, VA. I am 65 years old. I am a diabetic. At the time I had the sleeve procedure I weighed 251 pounds with a waist measurement of 42 inches. I was increasing my insulin daily to 130 units to maintain the proper control of my diabetes. I have lost about 50 pounds, am now down to a size 36 waist and 43 units of insulin. In my book that is truly a success story!

You may ask why haven't you lost more weight by this time? I have done this by design, I wanted to enjoy the process.

How is life after surgery? My Endocrinologist is happy with my blood sugar readings and the tighter control I have over my diabetes. I've gone from taking 8 different medications for my diabetes to 4 to give me long-term protection for my kidneys. I take daily supplements to ensure I receive the proper vitamin nutrients. I'm drinking more water daily, reading labels not so much for carbs as for proteins. That was quite a change for me.

I retired from the US Air Force so I have time now to enjoy my freedom from the 10-12 hour workdays of the past. I have a Golden Retriever puppy, an 80 pound hairball of energy and we walk about 3-4 miles a day or an hour (whichever comes first). Additionally, I spend some time in Dr. Clark's gym working out.

Some mornings I'm glad to be alive but don't want to get out of bed because I feel so sore...that comes from being able to do more yard work and other things that I didn't feel like doing because of the excess weight I was carrying. I start the day with a light breakfast (never ate breakfast when I was working). Getting up early in the morning sure beats the alternative.

Going through this surgery was a good deal for me because it was the catalysis I needed to get in shape and start watching my dietary intake on a daily basis. I put on a pound or two if I get lazy and don't exercise because of the weather or because I have a busy day of fishing. I monitor my weight and blood pressure every morning when I get up... just a habit I've gotten into since surgery. I think it's a good thing to do because as Dr. Clark tells me... "The surgery is just a management tool, not the cure all."

Before

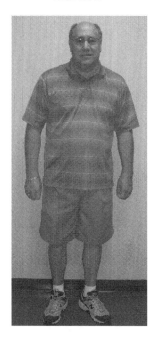

After

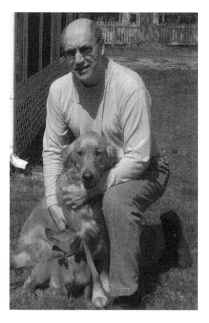

CHAPTER 16

WILL I NEED TO TAKE
VITAMINS AND SUPPLEMENTS?

Yes, you will need to take vitamins. Supplements are helpful but not a requirement. Actually, whether or not you have weight loss surgery, you should be taking vitamins. Supplements can be helpful as well, especially if you are trying to lose weight. You should also make sure your vitamins/supplements are pharmaceutical grade so that the quality of their content is monitored and guaranteed. The nutritional store at the Center for Weight Loss Success only carries such vitamins and supplements and our patients love them. To check out our inventory visit www.cfwls.com.

The common vitamins that will likely be recommended for you (may vary depending upon the surgeon) but usually include the following:

Multivitamins: Taking vitamins will be a lifelong commitment for all patients who have had weight loss surgery. In the beginning, you should take two chewable complete multivitamins each day. At one month after surgery, you may be able to progress to taking two regular vitamins daily. We recommend two vitamins each day during the first year when your weight loss is most rapid. After the first year, you should continue to take one multivitamin a day. Women may want to consider a prenatal vitamin if pre-menopausal.

B-Complex: Usually around 1 month after surgery, we recommend that you also add one B-Complex vitamin each day (or even 2 per day). The B vitamins assist in muscle and nerve functioning and have been shown to increase a person's energy level over time. You cannot overdose on B vitamins. If you take in more than you need, you will simply rid yourself of any excess through your urine. It is common for B vitamins to cause your urine to be darker or a brighter yellow. This is normal. If you prefer, B-Complex is also available as an injection at the office as appropriate.

Essential Fatty Acids (EFA's): Take them – they're just good for you. By taking fish oil supplements, Omega-3 fatty acids are ingested in their biologically active form. They can be directly used to support cardiovascular, brain, nervous system, and immune function. The mini-soft gels are smaller and have a natural lemon flavor to prevent a "fishy" after taste. Our product is ultra-filtered to guarantee removal of mercury and other possible contaminants. Most people should take 2-4 soft gels per day. They are also helpful to prevent constipation.

Magnesium-Potassium: During weight loss your body will tend to waste both magnesium and potassium. Both of these minerals are essential to normal muscular and cardiovascular function. Magnesium is involved in over 300 biological reactions throughout the body. It can help prevent/treat fatigue. If you are prone to muscle cramps – you need to add this supplement. Typical doses are 1-4 tablets daily with food.

Rhonda's Opinion: *Yes, Yes – they are good for everyone!!*

CHAPTER 17

What Should I Do After Weight Loss Surgery to Guarantee My Results?

This is a great question and one that isn't asked often enough. Understandably, your initial focus is usually on researching the available surgical options. After that, your next focus tends to be who will perform your surgery, where your surgery will be performed and how much it will cost. Unfortunately, the focus doesn't usually turn to one of the most important considerations - what you need to do after surgery to get the best long-term results.

The reality is that everyone loses weight after weight loss surgery (particularly with the gastric bypass and sleeve gastrectomy procedures). It's exciting! It's rewarding! It's awesome! But…eventually…your weight loss slows down and you will plateau. Don't despair, with proper support and guidance, you can get through plateaus and the final plateau will ideally be somewhere just above your ideal body weight.

This occurs, especially if you use the time after surgery (particularly the first year) to not only lose weight, but learn how to modify your mindset and your lifestyle habits…for good! If you do this, your potential for true long-term success is exponentially increased. Remember, weight loss surgery is a tool to lose weight. If you don't fully understand how to properly use your tool, your results can be compromised. Instead, why not optimize your results? This is where your post-operative comprehensive program comes in. Don't skip this important aspect of your research process prior to surgery.

This may be disheartening to hear because you might think of weight loss surgery as a guarantee. Don't get me wrong, I see success each and every day and it is truly amazing! However, weight loss surgery is not a magic bullet. Long-term success requires long-term changes. Don't worry though. With proper comprehensive support, this process is not only rewarding and fulfilling, it is actually fun!

So...What should you do after weight loss surgery to guarantee your results? This was reviewed somewhat in Chapter 10 but I am going to expand this explanation. I will begin with identifying the most common things you *should* be doing and then I will take a slightly different approach and share with you *the five most common culprits to poor or slower weight loss or eventual weight re-gain.*

In addition to the actions described in Chapter 10, your post weight loss surgery steps to success should include:

1. Don't miss your post-operative visits with your surgeon. It is important for him/her to monitor your recovery and progress. Sometimes people avoid their visits because either they are feeling so great, they don't think they need to be seen or they are struggling and too embarrassed to see their surgeon due to a perceived sense of failure. Unfortunately, this is the time you REALLY need to come in for your visits. If you feel great, you can confirm your progress and celebrate even more. If you are doing well, your surgeon WANTS to see you and celebrate with you as well. If you are struggling, your surgeon WANTS to see you to help you identify the reason(s) why you are struggling. It is best if this occurs as early as possible so you can take necessary actions to get back on track as soon as possible. *You are not alone* and recommendations can usually be determined quickly. You can leave with a plan in hand and

the confidence you need to master the use of your new tool and get back on your path to success.

2. Don't miss any scheduled visits with your primary care provider. This is particularly important if you are on any medications that need to be adjusted as you lose weight (i.e. hypertension and diabetes medications).

3. Don't miss any scheduled visits with your team of weight loss coaches. Included in comprehensive programs such as the one offered at the Center for Weight Loss Success, you will also be coached regularly by a dietician, weight loss coach and/or personal trainer. These professionals help you navigate the specific barriers or situations that may impede your optimal progress. They will also keep you on track and guide you through this life changing experience. In addition, your team loves to help you celebrate your success and assist you to avoid pitfalls and create new habits that keep you headed in the right direction.

4. Make the most of the educational materials provided to you before and after surgery. At the Center for Weight Loss Success, you receive a comprehensive pre-operative and post-operative learning series called Weight Management University for Weight Loss Surgery™. This program is reviewed at your office visits and delivered to your doorstep each month for

the first 12 months after surgery. They arrive in the form of monthly modules that explain what to expect that month, what to expect the next month, success stories, recipes and educational materials explaining what you need to know. They also include information regarding nutrition, metabolism, fitness and other topics that assist you to attain your optimal success. The modules are supported by DVD's, CD's and homework assignments that you will review at your monthly coaching visits. This comprehensive system is well received by patients. By the end of your first year after surgery, you will feel as if you have earned a new degree in weight loss surgery! No matter what learning method you prefer, all bases are covered so dive on in and enjoy!

5. Attend the support group provided by your experienced surgeon/center. These are generally offered in a group setting and often supplemented with online support as well.

6. Surround yourself with positive and supportive people who have healthy behaviors. Beware of saboteurs. There will usually be someone at work or at home who intentionally or unintentionally attempts to sabotage your new way of life. Sabotage comes in many forms. Here are a few strategies for dealing with the most common types:

- **Self-Sabotage:** Hard to admit, but sometimes we are

our own worst enemies. Do you have an internal dialogue that sounds like a tug of war between something you want to do and a rationalization as to why you can't possibly do that today (better known as excuses)? It all starts with a realistic goal, a realistic plan and realizing that you are in control of your own behavior. Try replacing the word "can't" with the word "won't" the next time that happens and your "self-talk" will begin to change!

- **Family/Friends:** You like to think they are all supportive but the reality is that those we count on the most for support are often the ones encouraging a "treat", "celebration", "one more bite" or those trigger foods that you can't say no to. The truth is that you are vulnerable right now and they need to understand your dedication to your goal. You may need to have a "heart-to-heart" asking for their support. Be assertive, keep your goals handy, put treats out of site or give them away, focus on activities rather than food events. At parties, focus on conversation and go in with a plan of attack you know you can stick to.

- **Vacations:** Time away should be a time to enjoy and relax. However, be careful about your sabotaging thoughts to "let loose", "do nothing" or "blow it out for the week". You can have fun in moderation, incorporate a new sport or activity, enjoy new foods (focus on protein, new vegetables or fruit) and feel great by working in a long walk, run or visit to the fitness center at that great resort!

• **Office Life:** Why is it that your office has to celebrate every event with cakes, cookies & donuts? Let your co-workers know you are trying to get healthier and welcome them to join you. Start a new office healthy thinking initiative. Avoid trips to the snack-laden break room and take your break outside. Make a point not to eat at your desk or if you have to, only bring things you know fit into your plan. Keep a stretch band or set of small weights at your desk to use. You could use eight different muscle groups in an eight-hour day!

• **Holidays/Parties:** We need to celebrate life! It can be done though without all of the focus being on food and/or alcohol (which diminishes our sense of control). Plan for the event ahead of time and don't go hungry. You will be less tempted. Plan on picking one or two special food items, giving yourself permission to sample what is there...you don't want to feel deprived. Keep your alcohol consumption absent or to a minimum and stay hydrated with water with a twist of lemon or lime. Hold your drink in your dominant hand to avoid picking at food and talk to others...it's harder to eat while you are talking.

You can overcome these problem areas! Make sure you identify what is risky for you so you can have a game plan to combat the situation(s). Don't prevent yourself from enjoying life but sometimes (especially early on in your weight loss until new habits are developed) it is easiest to limit exposure, make small strides, build your confidence and then celebrate your success!

Another way to look at how to achieve long-term success is to know and understand the most common reasons you might not get the results you desire and what to do about them. Below are *the five most common culprits to poor or slower weight loss or eventual weight re-gain:*

1. **Depression** – Emotional health is as important as physical health. Although depression is not a problem for most after surgery, it can be a significant deterrent to optimal weight loss. It is important to identify depression (admit that it is ok) and seek appropriate treatment so you can move on with your weight loss journey.

2. **Not Exercising** – I require each of you to complete a fitness evaluation with a personal trainer which is included with the program. The reason for this is because I believe some form of consistent exercise is essential for optimal success.

You should determine what form of exercise is right for you and begin your exercise plan before surgery. We cannot over-emphasize the importance of this factor. Although most find it difficult to begin an exercise plan, those that take that plunge never regret it. It can only enhance your weight loss experience and progress.

3. **Drinking High Calorie Liquids** – Many do not realize the excessive amount of sugar and calories contained in some liquids (i.e. Gatorade, Juice, Soda). As a result, you may "waste" calories on such liquids. This can significantly impede your weight loss. It is better to choose water, water with lemon, Fruit2O, Crystal Light or other low or no calorie drink options.

4. **"Grazing"** – After the first 2 months or so, you should have progressed to three meals per day with some higher protein snacks in between. If not, you may develop the habit of "grazing" or eating throughout the day. If this is the case, you tend to take in a significantly higher amount of calories throughout the day (more than what your body needs). This will slow down your weight loss and can potentially cause weight re-gain. Please guard yourself against such habits.

5. **Eating and Drinking at the Same Time** – When you eat and drink at the same time, the food is "washed through" the

stomach quickly. It is important to hydrate yourself by drinking a low/no calorie beverage approximately 30 minutes prior to eating. In this way, your hunger will be decreased. When you eat, you should not drink at the same time. As a result, your "pouch" will remain fuller for a longer period of time. Thus, you will remain satisfied for a longer period of time. Be sure to stop eating before you truly feel "full". It is a slow communication process from your stomach to your brain that indicates a feeling of fullness. Thus, you may overeat and realize it too late. This can be a very uncomfortable feeling.

So although you may be focusing on the surgery itself, you will be doing yourself a big favor by not neglecting your postoperative plan. Use these tips and don't forget to enjoy this journey of self-discovery.

Rhonda's Opinion: *Make yourself a priority and it will work.*

CHAPTER 18

WHAT QUESTIONS SHOULD I ASK WHEN TRYING TO FIND A QUALIFIED BARIATRIC SURGEON?

If you are considering weight loss surgery, you are likely quite savvy in your research and know what you are looking for. In fact most people research weight loss surgery for at least one year prior to deciding to have surgery and choosing which experienced surgeon will perform their procedure. This is actually refreshing to me and my professional team at the Center for Weight Loss Success. I welcome any and all questions and actually worry a bit if there are no questions. I will answer your questions with sincerity and honesty. This is very important because your relationship with your surgeon is for life and on-going support is critical to long-term success.

Below is a basic list of questions you should ask any bariatric surgeon under consideration. Although most are a standard part of your initial meeting and individualized consultation, they are important to know. You will likely have others so be sure to add them to the list prior to your individual consultation appointment.

- How many years have you been a bariatric surgeon?

- How many and what types of weight loss procedures have you performed and do you perform each year?

- Are you a board-certified surgeon?

- Are you a member of ASMBS (American Society for Metabolic & Bariatric Surgery)?

- Based on my personal health and weight, what surgery do you recommend for me?

- What are the advantages/disadvantages/risks of this procedure?

- Do you perform the surgery laparoscopically or open?

- Will you perform the procedure, or an assistant?

- Where will the surgery be performed?

- Is the hospital or clinic a Center of Excellence?

- What pre-op testing will be done?

- What post-op testing will be done?

- Do you have a comprehensive pre-operative and post-operative program including nutritional coaching, fitness, ongoing support groups, ongoing education and availability of a psychologist?

- What changes will I be expected to make with regards to diet and exercise?

- Do you have an insurance and/or financial coordinator available for patients?

- Do you have a dietician or nutritionist available for patients?

- Do you have a psychologist available for patients?

- Do you have a support group for patients?

- How are questions during non-office hours handled?

- What should my expected weight loss be?

- Ask for specific statistics regarding complications and

outcomes with your particular type of surgery. They should be willing to provide the information and not try to hide any negative results.

- Do you have patients who are willing to share their experiences with me?

If you can find a bariatric surgeon who is also experienced and/or board certified in bariatric medicine, that is an added bonus since they will also be equipped to assist you in losing weight prior to surgery. They also understand medical weight loss methodology that helps the further out you are from surgery. There are only a select few bariatric surgeons who are also board certified in bariatric medicine. I have chosen this route because it is my passion and I feel it provides me with the added knowledge to assist patients with or without surgery and also enhance their long-term success.

Your individualized consultation with your prospective surgeon should be thorough and informative. In addition to your surgeon, you will want to feel comfortable with the office staff and overall customer service experience. You are becoming a new member of their weight loss surgery family when you choose to have surgery. Your surgeon and his/her staff are your extended support system. They should also provide you with the opportunity to include your significant other each step of the way so they can also understand what to expect before, during and after surgery.

Rhonda's Opinion: *This is different for everyone. I looked at the experience and program offerings of the physician. With Dr. Clark it seemed like a no brainer.*

CHAPTER 19

WHAT QUESTIONS SHOULD I DISCUSS WITH MY PRIMARY CARE DOCTOR?

Particularly if you have a number of medical problems, your primary care practitioner and your bariatric surgeon will need to communicate openly throughout your pre-operative and post-operative phases of weight loss surgery. In addition, some insurance carriers require a letter from your primary care physician indicating that you are an appropriate candidate for weight loss surgery and/or "cleared" for surgery. If this is the case, the staff at your bariatric surgeon's office will be able to help you facilitate receiving such information prior to authorization for surgery.

Amazingly a number of people do not have a primary care provider. If this is the case for you, your surgeon will likely recommend that you find one. He/she will want to communicate your progress and have someone to refer you to in the event you have a medical problem unrelated to surgery and/or necessary medication changes as you lose weight following surgery.

Some questions you will want to discuss with your primary care provider include:

1. Are there any medical reasons that would prevent me from being an appropriate candidate for weight loss surgery?

2. Do you recommend any particular weight loss surgeon and the reason(s) why?

3. Are you able to provide my surgeon with any necessary documentation or clearance that might be required?

Most primary care practitioners are comfortable answering these questions and are used to working closely with an experienced local bariatric surgeon. Some may be limited in terms of who they are able to recommend due to required referral patterns within health systems. However, this is not generally the norm and the final decision is yours.

Rhonda's Opinion: *Will they miss you when you don't have to visit as often. :-)*

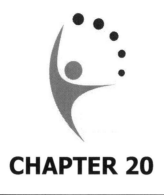

CHAPTER 20

HOW DO I FIND A QUALIFIED
WEIGHT LOSS SURGEON?

The search for a qualified weight loss surgeon can be completed in a number of ways. Some of the more common methods include:

1. Personal referral from someone you know

2. Referral from your primary care practitioner

3. Online search

4. Author/Expert Publication such as a journal or the book you are reading

5. Local marketing (i.e. radio, billboard, TV, newspaper or other publication)

Remember to ask the questions reviewed in Chapter 18. Evaluate the available options and select the surgeon, staff and program that will best fit you and your needs. This is a decision that requires careful consideration. Talking to someone who has already had surgery with the surgeon you are considering is often very helpful.

You will want to attend an on-site seminar with the surgeon (not just his/her assistant or office staff). This is a great way to get to know the surgeon, learn about the various procedures he/she performs, their particular outcomes, the comprehensive program they offer, get to meet their staff and learn more about your options. If you are unable to attend an on-site seminar, many surgeons also offer a comprehensive online webinar such as the one on our website at www.cfwls.com.

Rhonda's Opinion: *Find an experienced surgeon that has it all – you are worth it. I can't help but wholeheartedly recommend Dr. Clark! My life is changed forever and I am so happy.*

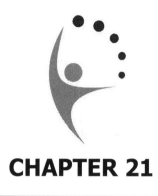

CHAPTER 21

What Can I Do If I Can't Find a Qualified Bariatric Surgeon or Comprehensive Follow-up Program in My Area?

If you cannot find a qualified bariatric surgeon or comprehensive follow-up program in your area, you will have to either compromise what you want and need or continue your search until you find the surgeon/program that will meet and/or exceed your expectations.

A few experienced surgeons offer a travel program for surgery. At the Center for Weight Loss Success, we offer such a program for appropriate surgical candidates. Not only does the program include surgery with arguably the most experience bariatric surgeon in the United States who has performed nearly 4,000 weight loss procedures, but it also includes our comprehensive Weight Management University for Weight Loss Surgery™ program. In addition, it is one of the most affordable options available in the United States. You can learn more about it at www.cfwls.com.

The bottom line is that you have to be comfortable with your choice. We are fortunate to have many excellent bariatric surgeons in the United States. Your long-term success is the most important thing under consideration here. I hope this book has helped to inspire you, an.swer your questions and better prepare you for an amazing journey.

Only you know if this journey is something that is right for you. If we can be of further assistance in any way, please let us know at success@cfwls.com. If you desire additional information and would like to view helpful videos that address each of these questions, please visit our main website at www.cfwls.com or at www.MyWeightLossSurgerySuccess.com.

Rhonda's Opinion: *Travel to the surgeon/program of your choice – it's all worth it!*

Sara's Story

Dr. Clark and his staff have been both supportive and encouraging throughout my weight loss journey of 109 pounds after the sleeve procedure, because of them, I have become a new person both physically and mentally.

Before

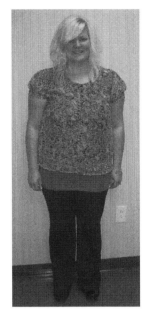

After

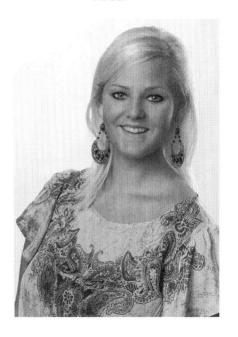

Supplemental Bonus

ACTION GUIDE CHECKLIST

The decision making process can be complex. This action guide checklist is intended to help you streamline this process. It contains a summary tool based upon the information provided in this book. You can use this checklist right away as you complete your research process to determine if weight loss surgery is the right decision for you. Educated decisions are generally the best decisions. You and your success is what matters most.

As you prepare, get a journal or notebook, you will find it helpful to document your research and questions. This will help to organize your thoughts and your resources in one place. Enjoy your journey along this path of discovery, decision and transformation leading to the most fulfilling, healthy and happy life possible.

✓ Read this book

✓ Get the videos that complement this book at www. MyWeightLossSurgerySuccess.com

✓ e-Mail your receipt to join-myweightlosssurgerysuccess@ instantcustomer.com for two bonus webinars by Dr. Clark (Optimizing Weight Loss after Weight Loss Surgery & Top 10 Dieting Mistakes and What to Do About Them)

✓ Determine Your BMI. In general, if you are utilizing insurance for weight loss surgery your BMI must be 35-39 with other significant, potentially life threatening health problems such as high blood pressure, diabetes or sleep apnea OR be 40 or greater. You *may* still be a candidate for weight loss surgery if you do not meet these criteria, but that would have to be determined with your bariatric surgeon based upon your specific situation.

✓ List the weight loss surgery option(s) you are interested

in pursuing along with their respective risks/benefits and common outcomes.

✓ Do some soul searching after reading this book to ensure that you feel motivated and committed to make the positive behavioral changes that must accompany weight loss surgery for optimal results. As Rhonda clearly states…you are worth it!

✓ Call your insurance agency and ask them if weight loss surgery is a covered benefit for your particular policy. Specifically ask them if your policy requires a "Ryder" for weight loss surgery and if so, if the Ryder is a part of your policy.

✓ Ask your insurance company what the requirements are for your policy in order to qualify for weight loss surgery (i.e. psychological clearance, your documented weight over the past 1 year etc…) These requirements vary by insurance company and policy.

✓ Find an experienced bariatric surgeon with a comprehensive pre-operative and post-operative program. Attend one of his/her seminars or view one of their online webinars.

✓ Schedule an individualized consultation with the surgeon(s) you are considering. Bring your list of questions with you. Get to know the office staff as well along with the surgery scheduler. The surgery scheduler should be able to clearly guide you through any requirements your insurance company may have.

✓ If insurance is not an option for you, talk with the surgeon and his/her staff regarding what package price options are available to you along with financing options as necessary.

✓ If you don't have a primary care practitioner, get one now.

✓ Enlist the support of your family as appropriate. Having someone at home supporting you each step of the way is not required but can be extremely helpful. This decision is yours. If you don't have a family member who will support you find a friend that will.

✓ Based upon your research and your experience with any surgeon(s) you are considering, begin the authorization or self-pay process if you feel weight loss surgery is the right decision for you.

✓ Obtain insurance authorization and/or commit to a comprehensive self-pay option for weight loss surgery.

✓ Actively participate in your surgeons pre-operative program by attending a support group meeting, completing any necessary medical clearances/documentation, and beginning your educational classes and coaching appointments that are a part of his/her comprehensive program. Include your significant other/support person if possible.

✓ Apply what you are learning in your life prior to surgery. Begin your weight loss journey prior to surgery and begin to integrate the actions discussed in Chapter 8 of this book.

✓ Organize your life (work and home) so that you will be able to focus on YOU after surgery. This is not selfish; it is the right thing to do. You will thank me for this advice.

✓ Work with your primary care practitioner to optimize any health problems that you may have (i.e. have your blood sugar levels and blood pressure under control)

✓ The day(s) prior to surgery, pamper yourself and meditate a bit (if appropriate for you) to make sure you are not only physically ready for surgery but emotionally as well. Believe it or not, in medicine, a positive attitude goes a long way as well as excellent medical/surgical care.

✓ Attend all of your scheduled appointments – you need to make yourself a priority.

✓ Follow your surgeons instructions before and after surgery.

✓ After surgery, attend all of your surgeon appointments, coaching appointments, fitness appointments, educational classes/webinars and fitness classes (once released by your surgeon to do so). The more you are up, moving and focusing on your new lifestyle behaviors, the sooner you will feel better and see results.

✓ If your surgeon provides a comprehensive program such as Weight Management University for Weight Loss Surgery™, devour the information, ask questions and integrate these new healthy habits into your life. If you are having difficulty, that is ok – be sure to meet with your surgeon and/or his expert staff so they can help you navigate your way to optimal success.

✓ Be an example for others. Weight loss surgery is a personal decision but it is a wonderful option for people who have >50 pounds to lose and desire the positive changes that comes with successful long-term weight loss.

✓ If you have any questions at all, please do not hesitate to contact us at success@cfwls.com or (757) 873-1880. Your success is our goal.

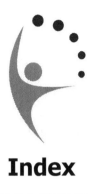

Index

[1] http://www.cdc.gov/PDF/Frequently_Asked_Questions_ About_Calculating_Obesity-Related_Risk.pdf

[2] http://www.nih.gov/news/pr/mar2005/nia-16.htm)

[3] Bariatric Surgery for Severe Obesity. Consumer Information Sheet. National Institute of Diabetes and Digestive and Kidney Diseases. March 2008. http://win.niddk.nih.gov/ publications/gastric.htm

4 http://www.cdc.gov/healthyweight/assessing/bmi/adult_bmi/english_bmi_calculator/bmi_calculator.html

5 http://asmbs.org/benefits-of-bariatric-surgery/

6 Obesity Action Coalition website:

www.obesityaction.org/obesity-treatments/bariatric-surgery

Fact Sheet: Why it makes sense to provide treatment for obesity through bariatric surgery.

18893289R00080

Made in the USA
Charleston, SC
26 April 2013